T0212322

Nursing Care of Adoption
and Kinship Families

Karen J. Foli, PhD, RN, FAAN, is an associate professor and the director of the PhD in nursing program at Purdue University, School of Nursing, West Lafayette, Indiana. She received her undergraduate degree from Indiana State University, her master's degree from Indiana University School of Nursing, Indianapolis, and her PhD in communications from the University of Illinois, Urbana/Champaign. She is a fellow in the American Academy of Nursing and has received numerous teaching awards, including the Charles B. Murphy Outstanding Undergraduate Teaching Award from Purdue University.

For the past 15 years, Dr. Foli's research program has focused on the transitions and needs of nontraditional social units: adoptive and kinship families. Through her research in the area of parental postadoption depression, Dr. Foli has described and tested a mid-range theory of postadoption depression and articulated the profiles of parents who struggle with depressive symptoms before and after placement; she has published her findings in nursing and interdisciplinary journals. Dr. Foli is a member of the *Adoption Quarterly* editorial board and has authored or coauthored three additional health-related books, including one specifically about adoption, *The Post-Adoption Blues: Overcoming the Unforeseen Challenges of Adoption*. Coauthored with John R. Thompson, MD, the book focuses on helping adoptive parents recognize and overcome challenges related to the placement of a child.

Nursing Care of Adoption and Kinship Families

A Clinical Guide for Advanced Practice Nurses

KAREN J. FOLI, PHD, RN, FAAN

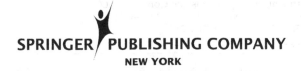

SPRINGER PUBLISHING COMPANY
NEW YORK

Springer Publishing Company, LLC
11 West 42nd Street
New York, NY 10036
www.springerpub.com

Acquisitions Editor: Elizabeth Nieginski
Senior Production Editor: Kris Parrish
Composition: S4Carisle Publishing Services

ISBN: 978-0-8261-3358-8
e-book ISBN: 978-0-8261-3359-5

16 17 18 19 20/5 4 3 2 1

The author and the publisher of this Work have made every effort to use sources believed to be reliable to provide information that is accurate and compatible with the standards generally accepted at the time of publication. Because medical science is continually advancing, our knowledge base continues to expand. Therefore, as new information becomes available, changes in procedures become necessary. We recommend that the reader always consult current research and specific institutional policies before performing any clinical procedure. The author and publisher shall not be liable for any special, consequential, or exemplary damages resulting, in whole or in part, from the readers' use of, or reliance on, the information contained in this book. The publisher has no responsibility for the persistence or accuracy of URLs for external or third-party Internet websites referred to in this publication and does not guarantee that any content on such websites is, or will remain, accurate or appropriate.

Library of Congress Cataloging-in-Publication Data

Names: Foli, Karen J., author.
Title: Nursing care of adoption and kinship families : a clinical guide for
   advanced practice nurses / Karen J. Foli.
Description: New York : Springer Publishing Company, [2017] | Includes
   bibliographical references and index.
Identifiers: LCCN 2016041438| ISBN 9780826133588 | ISBN 9780826133595 (e-book)
Subjects: | MESH: Nursing Care | Foster Home Care | Child Care | Adoption |
   Family Relations | Needs Assessment | United States
Classification: LCC HV875 | NLM WY 100 AA1 | DDC 362.73/3--dc23 LC record available at
https://lccn.loc.gov/2016041438

Printed in the United States of America by McNaughton & Gunn.

To families, no matter what the size, shape, or color, and to my father, Reno Foli, who loved such a family.

Contents

□ □ □ □

Section III: Position Statement Regarding Adoption
   and Kinship Nursing

Foreword

□ □ □ □

This is a landmark book that should have a global readership. For far too long, adoption and kinship families have not received the attention that they so sorely need. Karen Foli has written a text for which clinicians and academics have long been waiting—it will bring visibility to the welfare of adoption and kinship families. The material in this book is well researched, sensitively delivered, and essential for any clinician attending to adoption and kinship families.

The book acknowledges that the typical family—male and female parents with a boy and girl offspring—no longer reflects our society. Nontraditional families, such as adoptive and kinship families, are well entrenched in our society. In this book, Karen Foli draws clinicians' attention to the unique, heterogeneous families that have experienced relinquishment and acceptance of parenting by persons who have not given birth to the children and have no direct biological ties. With combined expertise and caring, Dr. Foli presents clinicians with much-needed resources. She carefully addresses the unique challenges of advanced practice nurses who are in a position to support adoptive and kinship families.

This well-researched book systematically focuses on each person involved in adoptive and kinship parenting. First, clinicians learn about the historical, cultural, and legal perspectives. Next, advanced practice nurses learn what is needed to deliver excellent nursing care to the birth parents, the adoptive parents, the child who is adopted, kinship parents, birth parents of kinship children, kinship children, and, lastly, special cases of foster care, assisted reproductive technology, commercial surrogacy, and human trafficking.

This book is not just a scholarly text but also a valuable manual and therefore represents a particular pinnacle of achievement within this field. I have little doubt this book will be read by many advanced practice nurses and other clinicians who will find the information in it extremely valuable and its message inspirational. The book will have an incredible impact on the care delivered by advanced practice nurses to make a significant difference in the lives of adoptive and kinship families. Thank you, Karen Foli, for your enduring passion for improving the lives of these long-forgotten families.

Cheryl Tatano Beck, DNSc, CNM, FAAN
Board of Trustees Distinguished Professor
School of Nursing
University of Connecticut
Storrs, Connecticut

Preface

□ □ □ □

She was about 9 years old and had been born with spina bifida. The little girl was one of my first patients in my nursing career, and a person whom I will always remember. Thirty-five years ago, I was entering into my community health clinical rotation as a student nurse, and was assigned to a family that also cared for foster children. But Grace, the little girl with long brown hair and glasses that made her eyes seem enormous, was my primary patient and a birth child to the foster mom, Patricia. Patricia and I talked about her other children and foster kids, and her husband, who worked in the local glass factory. Patricia was a petite woman with short, soft brown, curly hair and gentle blue eyes. The etchings of time around her eyes seemed more obvious when she smiled, but it was worth seeing and hearing her laugh. Yet there was a pervasive sadness around her, especially when she looked at Grace and knew that her daughter was vulnerable and always would be.

One day, to complete the family interview that was required, she said we could talk at the local café in a nearby strip mall. She had taken in an infant and knew the baby would be placed soon. The baby went into a stroller, and we walked to the small restaurant, where she ordered a piece of pie and a cup of coffee. The other children were at school, and she explained to me how she often would take about a half hour in the afternoon to come here and think. At the time, I thought how silly that was and what a waste of time. I simply did not have the insight and compassion to understand how resilient this woman was, how wise her behaviors were, and how these habits benefited her family and her ability to be present as a parent.

As a foster parent, she must have seen children come and go. She loved them, and then saw them leave for a new family. Other grief and loss colored her facial expressions. She must have known that her own daughter's future was uncertain. Grace suffered from frequent urinary tract infections. An additional worry was that the father, Patricia's husband, had been irritable lately. Stumbling in, by some miracle, I was able to discover during a visit at Grace's school that unsanitary conditions during her urinary catheterizations were the cause of the chronic infections. The school nurse instituted a new protocol for Grace's catheterizations to prevent contamination and break in sterile technique. During my rotation, I also discovered that the father suffered from hypertension, for which he was placed on medication by his physician. I counseled him regarding his diet and potassium levels. As the semester was at an end, I hoped that I was leaving the family with a fraction of what they had given to me. At the close of the last visit, Grace's mother gave me a present: a beautiful crocheted pink and gray blanket. My heart was touched, and I felt that maybe, just maybe, I could be a good nurse one day. I still have that blanket—it is upstairs in my linen closet—and its colors remind me of the myriad emotions that emanate from this world of taking care of children to whom we may not have given birth.

The grayness of seeing a child who has been damaged by cruelty and ignorance; the pewter-colored feeling of a birth mother grieving over relinquishment of her child; the shadow of a grandmother offering a bottle to a baby born with symptoms of drug withdrawal; the iron black color of adoptive parental depression—each certainly is an aspect of nontraditional families. Yet there is also the pink color of unconditional love; the yellow of healing a child who can now feel safe enough to attach to a parent; the rose-shaded knowledge that society is better because of sacrifice and selflessness; and the lavender hue of forgiveness and compassion— these, too, are facets of these families and found in the blanket that this mother gave to me. This book is about these families and the incredible difference that advanced practice nurses (APNs) can make in their lives.

The colors are representative of what I call the "adoption/kinship paradox"—the juxtaposition between loss and grief, renewal and healing. We know more about what we as humans need to attach and connect. We understand issues of identity and belonging. To really grasp these dynamics, the entire social unit needs to be considered, as well as the lives that are forever changed when a birth child is in the care of others. Although I believe the loss and grief must be recognized, healing and joy should be as well. And last, there is something incredibly human in our imperfections, and it has been my experience that parenting brings our imperfections into focus. When we cease to address these imperfections is when we stop living as moral human beings.

To be a family, and what that means in society today, is undergoing dramatic changes that reflect fluidity in definitions of spouse, children, and kin. The two-parent family with two children, a boy and a girl, no longer reflects our society with its diversity of genders and cross-ethnic members. As one becomes more aware of the presence of nontraditional families— such as adoptive and kinship families—one begins to see them within the fabric of society. It is as if this heightened sensitivity enables one to see through an additional set of lenses, and suddenly, adoptive and kinship families are seemingly everywhere.

Similarly, as nurses we do not often see ourselves as health care providers for adoptive or kinship families. Yet I have encountered many nurses who have cared for these individuals and families with—and without—the knowledge and insights that emanate from the cultural and social structures of adoption and kinship families. Through years of experience and research, I have come to realize that this care is special and specialized, and these are the reasons I decided to write this book. If there were ever populations that needed holistic care, they are nontraditional units such as adoptive and kinship families. And nurses are increasingly in positions to render such care through advanced practice opportunities.

Let us start by defining "adoption" and "kinship families." Legally, adoption is a process whereby birth parents' rights are terminated and adoptive parents are given legal permission to care for the child(ren) on a permanent basis. Thus, a triad is created, an adoptive triad composed of the birth parents (also called "first/birth parents"), the individual who is being adopted, and the adoptive parent(s). Statistics of adoptions can be elusive because estimates for annual numbers of adopted children are generated from state court records, the Adoption and Foster Care Analysis and Reporting System (AFCARS), and the U.S. Department of State's Bureau of Consular Affairs. The 2010 census revealed that 2,072,312 children or 2.3% of all children in the

United States are adopted (U.S. Census, 2010), with approximately 2 million adoptive parents caring for them (Jones, 2009).

Kinship parents differ in several ways. First, kinship parents are close family and friends who have assumed the care of the child on a permanent or temporary basis. There may be several generations of the family living in one home with several identified caregivers. However, some kin caregivers, often grandparents, elect to legally adopt their grandchildren and thus become adoptive parents. Across the country, states are relying on kinship care, rendered by extended family members and close friends, for the 2.7 million children who have been removed from their birth parents' care (Annie E. Casey Foundation, 2012). This book addresses all three members of these triads or triangles of family, and offers particular insights into their needs through the use of cases and analyses of those family units.

Adding these millions of individuals together, we have, conservatively, 8 to 9 million people (birth, adoptive, and kinship parents, and children/individuals who are adopted or cared for by kinship parents). Therefore, there are a significant number of people living in the United States who need health care providers who understand the contexts of their families, which include a wide scope of issues related to nursing care. Examples include infectious diseases, vitamin deficiencies, attachment and bonding, acute and chronic illnesses, caregivers' legal right to consent to treatment of a minor, and nonbirth mothers' decisions to induce lactation for an adopted infant. Complex interfaces with populations, groups, communities, and individuals color these nontraditional families. This text guides APNs through these contexts.

Although adoption and kinship families are found globally, this discussion focuses on the practices within the United States. Stepfamilies and traditional surrogates are also excluded from this text because there is a permanent, primary caregiver who is a birth parent in the home. We concentrate on those unique, heterogeneous families that are characterized by a relinquishment and an acceptance of parenting from individuals who did not give birth to the children and have no direct biological ties.

The readers of this book are APNs who work with adoption and kinship families— certified nurse-midwives, pediatric nurse practitioners, adult-gerontology nurse practitioners, family nurse practitioners, psychiatric mental health nurse practitioners, clinical nurse specialists, or clinical leaders (note that there is an assumption that APNs hold certification credentials in their areas of expertise). Areas of practice may be in community/public health, mental health, corrections, school nursing, and in acute and primary care areas. Educators of advanced practice courses may integrate this guide with the existing textbooks in courses such as nursing care of the childbearing family, pediatric nursing, psychosocial/mental health nursing, acute and chronic health, health promotion courses, gerontology courses (kinship parents are often older adults), and public/community health nursing.

With this guide, the nursing profession will be able to fully collaborate with other disciplines such as medicine and social work that have discussed and studied adoptive and kinship families for many decades. To strengthen the profession and consolidate this knowledge, two major goals to be accomplished through this book are:

1. **To change nursing's current thinking about adoption and kinship triads.** The primary purpose of this clinical guide is to inform nurses who care for members of the adoption and kinship triads with current, best clinical practices. The book is also designed to change the current view of adoption and kinship care. I have spoken to nurses and their interest is keen, yet they are apt to defer to other professionals to deliver care to triad members or they feel a sense of discomfort, knowing that there is little information surrounding nontraditional families, and they are unsure where to find such information. Despite hesitations, my research findings support the fact that nurses care for members of these triads in multiple settings. *Unfortunately, APNs and graduate student nurses have little clinical guidance that is specific to these populations.* I have also found that there is a lack of curricular content in undergraduate and graduate nursing programs to educate new nurses and APNs on best practices related to these populations. With this guide, nurses no longer have to continue to rely on intuition and can feel confident through evidence-based practice when rendering care.

2. **To disseminate knowledge to improve care rendered by nurses.** This book is a fount of knowledge and insight for those APNs who interface with adoptive and kinship triad members (birth parents, adoptive/kinship parents, and individuals who are adopted) across multiple health care settings. Each of the triad members is included

in this needed book that serves practicing nurses who wish to expand their clinical knowledge or as a clinical guide in many nursing courses. As professionals, we are called on to be holistic caregivers. Now more than ever, such humanistic care is needed by so many. This guide approaches these family social units as a whole with consideration of cultural preferences, health disparities, and issues of gender, class, and race. This information will empower APNs to deliver services grounded in evidence and patient-centered care.

Your Narrative

Finally, many of you have firsthand knowledge and may be part of an adoptive or kinship family. You may recognize elements of your situation or a family member's situation in these pages. Over the years, I have learned of many nurses—perhaps because of the fabric of who we are and what we do—who are members of such triads. Circumstances change, and we may find ourselves in families with a configuration we never anticipated, or we are experiencing feelings of loss that we are still processing. Or some of you may have planned and waited for years to expand your family through adoption. My narrative includes being a member of the adoption triad (adoptive mother), a researcher in the area of adoption and kinship families, and a cofacilitator in a trauma-informed parenting class for rural-dwelling kinship parents. These stories are important, and I hope that our personal narratives will enlighten us and, combined with knowledge, allow us to become providers of quality nursing care to adoption and kinship families.

Karen J. Foli

Acknowledgments

□ □ □ □

Books are never easy to write—although I love doing so. Writing hundreds of pages seems like a monumental undertaking, and, in some respects, it is. This book, however, was a labor of purpose: to consolidate knowledge surrounding the health care needs and social contexts of adoptive and kinship families so that advanced practice nurses' patient-centered assessments and interventions are of optimal quality and effectiveness. When you read these pages, I hope you will frequently say, "I didn't know that!" and provide informed, effective care as a result.

I believe that adoption and kinship nursing is a specialty area that deserves its own scope and standards of practice.

Although writing can be isolating, books are not written in isolation. Many people contributed to this book by offering emotional and instrumental support, and by advising on policies and practices from both an adoption and from an advanced practice nursing perspective. My colleagues and supporters represent a mix of friends, collaborators, and colleagues, many of whom are advanced practice nurses: Jenny Coddington, Melanie Braswell, Patricia Moisan-Thomas, Rhonda Moravec, Janet Thorlton, Jill Lintner, Susan Kersey, Nancy Edwards, Pam Karagory, Kristen Kirby, Becky Walters, Janelle Potetz, and Jan Davis. I would also like to thank Kathy Stagg, MSW, LCSW, The Villages; Sarah Horton-Bobo, MA, director of Post Adoption Support and Education, Bethany Christian Services; and Susan Livingston Smith, LCSW, emerita professor of social work, Illinois State University; all of whom were so helpful in my understanding of the complexities of adoption, the child welfare system, and foster care. Also, my extended family members, who cheered me on, are to be recognized: Adele Foli, Leanne and Bill Malloy, Margaret and Mark Conway, and Katherine Malloy.

When researching my book on postadoption blues in 2002, I reached out to Cheryl Beck and was grateful for her generosity and willingness to help a fellow nurse, albeit a stranger, who wanted to draw attention to the challenges faced by adoptive parents. Since then, Cheryl has been a mentoring presence, and her consistent kindness has been an important source of support. She graciously introduces the reader to this work (see her Foreword), for which I am grateful.

Elizabeth Nieginski, executive editor, and Rachel Landes, assistant editor, at Springer Publishing deserve so much gratitude. Elizabeth's vision for this book and her insight into the gap it fills in the nursing profession have been invaluable. Her advocacy to bring it to the nursing profession deserves recognition and respect. I am grateful to Rachel, whose professional communications and hard work helped to secure permissions for use of materials, as well as to shape and refine the chapters.

I thank my family, John, Ben, Peter, and Annie, who give me purpose and help me strive to be a better person. My husband and soulmate, John, gave me tireless encouragement during my moments of doubt and fatigue, and because of his steadfast loyalty, I was able to give this work my very best efforts. I want to specifically acknowledge my children: Ben, my older son, whose bravery and earnestness keep me grounded; Peter, whose honor and faith offer me values to be proud of; and Annie, whose forthrightness and affection warm my heart. They are truly gifts to my soul.

This book would not be possible without the nontraditional families whose sacrifices and joys continue to be sources of inspiration. My goal is to honor each member of the adoption and kinship triads and, through the information on the following pages, enhance and optimize the care they receive from advanced practice nurses in a wide variety of clinical settings.

I

Overview of Adoption and Kinship Families

Introduction

□ □ □ □

What do you know about adoption and kinship care? Do you have the skills to appropriately manage the care of these families? Perhaps the more important question is: How do you *feel* about these nontraditional families? What are your beliefs toward parents of the same sex raising children? Or birth parents who have abused and neglected their children? Or children who act out inappropriately because of past trauma? Many of us are influenced by media presentations that tend to depict individuals who are part of adoption and kinship triads as somehow lesser or more flawed than mainstream society. Do you believe that White parents should adopt Black or biracial children? Should all birth records be unsealed so that individuals who are adopted can seek out their birth parents—with or without their consent? These are challenging questions that need to be answered with accurate knowledge and honest reflection.

These and other issues create new conversations and additional ethical questions about the modern face of families in our society. Nurses, whether or not they have considered this, have an ethical responsibility to be aware of how to deliver quality and safe care to these nontraditional families.

KNOWLEDGE, SKILLS, AND ATTITUDES

Knowledge, skills, and attitudes (KSAs)—these three components are critical to graduate-level Quality and Safety Education in Nursing (QSEN) as outlined by the American Association of Colleges of Nursing (2012; see Exhibit A). Competencies at the graduate level in nursing include six areas, and each of these areas pertains to caring for adoption and kinship triads.

EXHIBIT A

DEFINITIONS OF QSEN COMPETENCIES

Quality Improvement (QI): Use data to monitor the outcomes of care processes and use improvement methods to design and test changes to continuously improve the quality and safety of health-care systems.

Safety: Minimize risk of harm to patients and providers through both system effectiveness and individual performance.

Teamwork and Collaboration: Function effectively within nursing and interprofessional teams, fostering open communication, mutual respect, and shared decision-making to achieve quality patient care.

Patient-Centered Care: Recognize the patient or designee as the source of control and full partner in providing compassionate and coordinated care based on respect for patient's preferences, values, and needs.

Evidence-Based Practice (EBP): Integrate best current evidence with clinical expertise and patient/family preferences and values for delivery of optimal health care.

Informatics: Use information and technology to communicate, manage knowledge, mitigate error, and support decision making

Source: AACN (2012)

Quality Improvement

Often, processes in managing the care of these special populations is lacking because most advanced practice nurses (APNs) need to acquire a knowledge base and the skills to manage the unique dynamics of adoption and kinship triads. Improving existing or current organizational policies, maintaining referral lists of adoption-competent mental health and medical professionals, and continuing education in trauma-informed care are examples of contributions to quality improvement (QI) in care. Often, nurses assume that these families comprise a small minority of the patients but a closer examination of this assumption is warranted with concurrent data collection processes put in place. Process flow maps of services and verification of care coordination between agencies and patient-centered medical home services may be part of a QI plan.

Nursing organizations whose members interface with adoptive and kinship families are provided in Exhibit B. Working within these various nursing organizations is important to increase awareness of nontraditional families' health care needs and to advocate for federal and state policies that support these families. This perspective, that many nursing organizations connect with members of these families, shifts our thinking from how we *provide* services to how individuals *receive* services.

EXHIBIT B

NURSING ORGANIZATIONS WHOSE MEMBERS INTERFACE WITH ADOPTIVE AND KINSHIP FAMILIES

- *American Nurses Association*
- *American Academy of Colleges of Nursing*
- *Emergency Nurses Association*
- *National League for Nursing*
- *National Association of Neonatal Nurses*
- *Association of Women's Health, Obstetric and Neonatal Nurses*
- *National Association of School Nurses*
- *National Association of State School Nurse Consultants*
- *American Psychiatric Nurses Association*
- *International Association of Forensic Nurses*
- *Home Health Nurses Association*
- *The Visiting Nurses Associations of America*
- *International Nurses Society on Addictions*

(continued)

EXHIBIT B *(continued)*

Advanced Practice Nurse Organizations:

- ☐ American Association of Nurse Practitioners
- ☐ American College of Nurse Midwives
- ☐ Canadian Association of Advanced Practice Nurses
- ☐ Gerontological Advanced Practice Nurses Association
- ☐ American Academy of Nurse Practitioners
- ☐ American College of Nurse Practitioners
- ☐ Association of Faculties of Pediatric Nurse Practitioners
- ☐ National Association of Certified Professional Midwives
- ☐ National Association of Nurse Practitioners in Women's Health
- ☐ National Association of Pediatric Nurse Practitioners
- ☐ National Conference of Gerontological Nurse Practitioners
- ☐ National Organization of Nurse Practitioner Faculties
- ☐ American Academy of Emergency Nurse Practitioners.

Safety

I have spoken with many individuals whose lives have been affected by adoption and kinship arrangements. Several of them have expressed how damaging the care from health care professionals can be when the caregiver is unaware of the special needs of these heterogeneous groups. Stereotypes, assumptions, and a lack of familiarity with best evidence affect safety in the delivery of care. Being skillful in trauma-informed care is critical to an accurate assessment and treatment plan. Avoiding generalizations, consuming evidence in peer-reviewed journals, and a strong referral base can also improve safe care.

There are also significant safety issues from the provider's perspective as children are removed from homes due to maltreatment (neglect and abuse), unregulated custody transfers (see Chapter 4), and running away or aging out of foster care, exposing children and young adults to human trafficking. As frontline care providers in primary care, APNs will need to assess for such neglect and abuse and report it. (note that federal law requires nurses and health care practitioners to report abuse and neglect [42 U.S. Code § 13031—Child Abuse Reporting].) For adoptive parents, depressive symptoms and issues of bereavement carry higher risks of negative outcomes for children (Pemberton et al., 2010; Tully, Iacono, & McGue, 2008).

Teamwork and Collaboration

Health care management of these families, including birth parents and siblings, needs to occur within the context of a team of collaborating professionals. Some of the key individuals may be outside of what we traditionally consider, such as adoption agency staff and facilitators, community mental health professionals, and professionals in the criminal justice system. They may also include Court Appointed Special Advocate (CASA) volunteers, those who speak on behalf of children's needs to the court (National CASA Association, 2015), child protective services/department of children and family services, support groups, and case workers all of whom remind us of the vulnerabilities of these families. Collaborators also include health care staff from international adoption clinics, which are primarily found in major universities across the country.

Social workers are often the first professional group to become involved with adoption and now oversee many kinship placements. However, nurses may actually be the first point of contact and are present in times of crisis, vulnerability, and, in many cases, on an ongoing basis for health-related needs as primary care providers. Physicians will be important team members. The American Academy of Pediatrics (AAP) has a special body, the Council on Foster Care, Adoption, and Kinship Care (COFCAKC), which was formed in 2011 when the Section on Adoption and Foster Care (founded in 2000) merged with relevant parts of the Committee on Early Childhood, Adoption, and Dependent Care. Physicians may specialize in "adoption medicine," experts in the medical needs of children who have been adopted, especially those from a developing country. These physicians will often review videotapes given to preadoptive parents from foster care homes and orphanages around the world. They will view these tapes and offer their opinions on potential health risks or educate on apparent health problems. The AAP has several on the assessment and health care management of children and adolescents in foster care (AAP, 2005, 2013). These resources are valuable to APNs in the pediatric setting as they provide and navigate services for triad members and, when necessary, refer care to colleagues.

Child and adolescent psychologists and psychiatrists and pediatric developmental specialists will also be consulted in evaluating and treating children and adolescents. Between 2000 and 2010, there has been a 60% increase in the number of emotionally disturbed children who have been placed in out-of-home (OOH) care and a 36% increase in the number of children in OOH care who have suffered from multiple maltreatment (as opposed to single maltreatment; Conn et al., 2013). These troubling statistics reflect significant health care needs, with an emphasis on mental health services, and implications for APNs as triage and treatment are offered.

For children who are medically fragile, are developmentally delayed, or suffer from infectious diseases and other medical problems, specialists will need to be consulted. These include infectious disease specialists, occupational and physical therapists, as well as audiologists and speech-language pathologists/therapists. Medical supply professionals may need to be called upon to provide equipment for medically fragile children as in-home care is planned. Pediatric pharmacists will also be part of the team when infants and children present with complex health care needs, as in cases of prenatal exposure to alcohol and other drugs.

Gerontologists may be important consultants when caregiver burden affects the health status of kinship parents, who may be in the seventh and eighth decades of life. One 69-year-old great grandmother confessed to long consideration before assuming the care—and legal adoption—of two young children. She worried about her health status and life expectancy with several chronic health conditions. APN referrals may include estate-planning attorneys to ensure that wills are current.

Patient-Centered Care

In addition to the Patient Protection and Affordable Care Act (2010), which supports patient-centered care and medical homes, the values espoused by patient-centered care infuse nurses' care for children, adolescents, and families who may be sewn together through adoption and kinship. Depending on the historical period (see Chapter 1), birth parents' rights have, in documented cases, been violated and dismissed. Lack of informed consent, rights to birth records, and misleading information have colored the practices of the past. Today, many birth parents remain disenfranchised, or even ostracized, uncertain of how others will perceive their decision to relinquish a child. Other birth parents are demonized if parental rights are involuntarily terminated. Their narratives of incarceration, substance use and abuse, and violence and neglect against their children are difficult to hear and understand. For many in society, the violation of societal mores, laws, and values supersedes and extinguishes their right to parent.

The world in which birth parents' rights are terminated or suspended have fueled many different perspectives, each influenced by a judgment of the best interest of the child. We know that in 2011, 70.4% of children were reunited with birth parents within 12 months of being removed from the home; however, what is concerning is that 11.8% reentered care less than 12 months from being discharged (Children's Bureau, 2011). With such interwoven issues, APNs will have multiple patients, and therefore the potential for ethical and moral conflicts in rendering patient-centered care.

Children and adolescents who have been in multiple placements before finding a permanent home may feel their rights and well-being have been ignored or subjugated as they belong to a "system." The abilities to have a voice, to feel safe, and to believe they have some control over their lives are critical themes the APN needs to understand. Feelings of distrust, an inability to attach, and anger over loss of control need to be countered with validation of feelings, nonjudgmental care, creation of a safe environment, respect for preferences, and a matter-of-fact approach. These thoughtful strategies mitigate the barriers and support optimal nurse–patient relationships.

The nonbirth parents who assume the care of adoptive and kinship children voluntarily enter into a parenting role; however, what that role entails may be more difficult and very different from what was expected. Understanding adoptive and kinship parents' transitions to parenting and the adjustments that need to be made, some born from caring for a child who has experienced trauma, APNs will need to listen, guide, refer, and demonstrate sensitivity toward these unique parents. Being a member of a nontraditional family is highly personalized: One individual may see a journey of growth and self-actualization; another may be reliving past trauma triggered by the child's maltreatment. Ethical principles such as justice, autonomy, fidelity, beneficence, and informed consent are critical aspects of APNs' care to these families.

Evidence-Based Practice

Adoption and kinship care, as objects of empirical examination, are not exclusive to any one profession. As such, a wide range of disciplines contribute to the evidence of best practices surrounding adoption and kinship care and include social work, psychology, psychiatry, pediatric medicine, sociology, genetics, human development and family studies, and nursing. Due to the multidisciplinary nature of the research, challenges exist in extracting this evidence into a cohesive body of knowledge. Additionally, while the research findings in adoption have been prolific, most of it has surrounded child outcomes. The child in adoption and kinship is viewed as the person of ultimate interest whose needs become the barometer of decisions made. Much less is known about birth parents, and kinship and adoptive parents' transitions to parenting.

Evaluation of postadoption/postplacement services is also an underdeveloped area receiving renewed interest. The adoption community—across disciplines—is consolidating in a call to better understand the needs of adoptive and kinship families after the child is home. Medical, psychological, financial, social, and instrumental support mechanisms are now being examined for impact toward achieving optimal permanent placements for the well-being of the entire family.

The evidence that is presented in this guide is based on policy and state laws, empirical research findings—both quantitative and qualitative—and credible sources, such as those found in peer-reviewed journals, government documents, and national adoption organizations. The National Survey of Adoptive Parents (NSAP; Vandivere, Malm, & Radel, 2009) is cited frequently as an appraisal that specifically assessed characteristics of adoptive families. Adoption policy and scope of practice for APNs share the fact that much is enforced at the state level. So while this guide provides information related to both adoption and advanced practice, be aware that states differ in adoption and kinship laws (e.g., how kinship is defined differs by state) as well as scope of practice for APNs.

Informatics

The Internet has transformed how adoption information is viewed and exchanged. How information is sealed, stored, retrieved, and disseminated is a core issue in adoption. As adoption is often overseen by the states, the access to birth records and original birth certificates vary by state law (American Adoption Congress, 2016); the issue of ownership of information is at the core of these discussions. Accurate birth records that reveal part of a person's past are viewed as rightful property by many individuals who have been adopted. This is also true for birth parents who have been denied access to such information once relinquishment occurred. Non-government-sponsored registries, such as the International Soundex Reunion Registry (2011–2012) and the Adoption Registry Connect (2015), have been created with hundreds of thousands of individuals seeking information about birth parents and children. States also sponsor registries, such as in Indiana where the Indiana Adoption Registry (Indiana Department of Health, 2015) posts information such as birth year, place of birth, and adoption agency involved. These registries serve individuals who seek to reunite with lost family members.

The issue of whether individuals desire to search and be located is of key concern when reunions are considered. There are "passive" or mutual-consent reunion registries, meaning that both parties must register for reunions to occur. The registry arranges for both parties' information to be shared. In contrast, an "active" registry will assist the individual in finding lost family members. Private registries and some states will actively search on behalf of individuals for a fee (Child Welfare Information Gateway, 2011). If an active search is pursued, one resource is Independent Search Consultants (2001), comprised of individuals who are certified in searching for family members in many states and some countries. Adoption attorneys may be enlisted to petition to open birth records, which may or may not be granted by a judge. Mutual consent may or may not be present. The National Council for Adoption (2014) specifically describes their stance on "Privacy in Adoption," advocating for a mutual consent bill since 1983, which would protect the rights of all adoption parties involved. Patient-centered care overlaps with informatics, creating a wide range of preferences in finding family members. From birth parents who confess, "Some of us don't want to be found," to a child longing to reconnect to a birth parent, APNs need to respect and understand the individuality of nontraditional family members.

The rights of adopted individuals to birth information versus the rights of family members' privacy can be a difficult balance. APNs' ethical beliefs should be examined and an understanding of all parties' rights should guide discussions with individuals who have been adopted and their siblings, as well as birth parents. As family history and connections are discovered, individuals may need support to process how their identities may be changed and reconceptualized.

Kinship parents present issues related to informatics in different ways. These families are aware of birth histories and other family information. However, they often decide to parent outside the child welfare system, instead preferring an informal arrangement across generations within the family. There are three types of kinship care arrangements. The first, informal kinship care, are private arrangements made between the birth parents and kin, such as grandparents, aunts and uncles, and close friends. In informal kinship arrangements, the child welfare and court systems are not involved with the placement. Resources that would be available to families who are connected to the child welfare system are not accessible to these families. Challenges with obtaining medical care and school services may be more complicated without any formal legal arrangements. The second form is voluntary kinship care, wherein relatives and kin take over the parenting of the child, but the state does not take legal custody. The parents may voluntarily relinquish care to kin or the court may order it, depending on the circumstances (Child Welfare Information Gateway, 2010).

The third type of arrangement is formal kinship care. In these cases, the child welfare system has legal custody of the child and the kinship parent has physical custody. Each state varies with regard to specific arrangements made between the child welfare departments and the kinship parents. These arrangements closely follow nonrelative foster parent arrangements. However, special circumstances exist for American Indian and Alaska Native children governed by the Federal Indian Child Welfare Act (P.L. 95-608), which states that tribes have the right to be involved with child welfare and placement of children (Child Welfare Information Gateway, 2010). Therefore, the information gathered and analyzed for kinship families is segmented and difficult to understand because of the variety of arrangements within these multigenerational families.

HOW THIS GUIDE IS ORGANIZED

APNs move forward with their professional lives in an independent and informed way to impact caring for others. Although many books have been written about adoption and kinship, this book is nursecentric and emphasizes the important roles and interventions provided by APNs to support adoptive and kinship triads. Members of the triad are highlighted in separate chapters. Each chapter begins with a brief overview that is specific to that triad member and includes the chapter's purpose and learning objectives. In-depth discussions of research findings follow. Case studies bring into focus actions by APNs as care is rendered and serve as springboards to promote continuing conversations and debates: What was done well in the case study? What could have been explored further? The case studies are not intended to be interpreted as reflecting the spectrum of situations in adoption and kinship families *nor are they prescriptions for care*. Rather, they exemplify important concepts that may be generalizable to these heterogeneous populations. Also note that any individuals or scenarios featured in the case studies are fictitious and used for instructional purposes only. There may be overlap between the parental and child categories. For example, a kinship parent may also be an adoptive parent. Similarly, an adopted child may also be a child being raised by kin. Descriptions of what APNs should assess for and potential interventions are offered, but again, are not necessarily comprehensive of all that the APN could and should do. Highlights of each chapter are listed, which help to emphasize key concepts. Questions to reflect on end the chapters and serve to stimulate insight into your own beliefs and behaviors toward these triads.

THEMES

The QSEN graduate competencies provide us with a glimpse of the multiple aspects of nursing care for these specific groups. There are also threaded themes to this clinical guide, which offer beliefs about APNs and their expanded roles in the nursing profession. Major themes threaded into this book are as follows:

☐ APNs affect the lives of individuals who have been touched by adoption and kinship care.

☐ A coherent body of knowledge specific to care rendered to non-traditional families by APNs is provided in this guide.

☐ By assimilating this knowledge, the nursing profession is propelled forward in delivering quality, patient-centered care for these unique families.

☐ This information applies to practicing APNs and APN students alike.

APNs Affect the Lives of Individuals Who Have Been Touched by Adoption and Kinship Care

The roles of social workers and physicians have been discussed in the existing literature, but far less has been described for APNs. Nurses are there when birth mothers are in labor; they are present in acute and long-term health facilities when family members need a holistic care provider. Nurses are there to provide physical assessments and counsel kinship and adoptive parents who may be struggling. In sum, APNs are there to provide education, support, referrals, and management to promote individual and family functioning. And when they do so, they affect individuals' health and their lives.

A Coherent Body of Knowledge Specific to Care Rendered to Nontraditional Families by APNs Is Provided in This Guide

Evidence pertaining to the practices of APNs is scattered across disciplines and across resources (e.g., empirical studies, books on adoption, and policy statements made by medical organizations). As previously discussed, the clinical settings in which nurses care for these clients are varied, from correctional facilities, psychiatric-mental health centers, and schools to primary care providers' clinics (women's health, older adult, and pediatric). Lastly, no single nursing organization is specifically designed to assist nurses in these areas. This text brings much needed information into a comprehensive, APN-focused guide.

The vocabulary of any specific discipline conveys a shortcut of meanings, subtexts that have the ability to convey shifting signs of significance and hegemony. At times, these words, such as those found in medical terminology, send efficient and precise meanings to the receiver. At other times, they alienate and subjugate the most important person in the health care context: the patient. In the adoption world, vocabulary is significant in several respects. For example, the words "give away" or "put up for adoption" communicate negative connotations in the decision-making process of birth parents. In contrast, to "relinquish a child" or "adoption plan" carries more positive and socially acceptable connotations. To "give away" a child implies a lack of value of that child, a lack of emotion, and an end point. Words create different realities and, therefore, different thoughts and actions. To enable APNs to participate in such conversations in an informed manner, a glossary of adoption terms that will increase awareness when delivering care to these triads has been provided at the end of this guide. Use of this vocabulary will support patient-centered, quality care.

By Assimilating This Knowledge, the Nursing Profession Is Propelled Forward in Delivering Quality, Patient-Centered Care for These Unique Families

The nursing profession, unlike medicine, does not offer specialty guidance on adoptive or kinship care. As previously described, the Council on Foster Care, Adoption, and Kinship Care, a body within the AAP, describes medical services for these patient groups (Mason, Johnson, & Prock, 2014). Similarly, the American College of Obstetricians and Gynecologists (2012) has issued a policy statement that delineates the role of the physician in adoptions. The American Society of Reproductive Medicine (2014) offers a fact sheet to those considering adoption after struggling with infertility. That being said, there have been pioneer nurse researchers, such as Teena

McGuinness, whose work in understanding children who have been adopted internationally has greatly informed nursing practice, and Carol Musil, PhD, RN, FAAN, FGSA, whose work with grandmother caregivers has contributed significantly to understanding the needs of this vulnerable population. But as a coherent whole, nursing, as a profession, is behind in addressing these important clinical areas.

This Information Applies to Practicing APNs and APN Students Alike

Educators may not be familiar with the unique needs of the adoptive and kinship triads. The outstanding feature of this book is to fill a major gap in nursing clinical practice and curricula across the United States by articulating the unique but common needs of members of these triads. Our role is not to offer advice to our patients when they are deciding whether to be a party in adoption or kinship families; the APNs' role is to be aware of the various elements that contribute to an informed decision. Following are select examples of content that is covered in this guide:

☐ Birth parents:
- The myriad reasons birth parents decide to or are legally ordered to relinquish their children to adoptive and kin parents
- Disenfranchised grief experienced by birth parents after relinquishing a baby or child
- The unique dynamics of having the grandparent take on the parenting of the relinquished child
☐ Adoptive/kinship parents:
- The unique contexts of adoption (history of infertility, adopting an older child, a child with unknown special needs, and bonding to the child)
- The societal barriers to "conspicuous families": same-sex partnered adoptive parents and parents who have adopted a child of a different race/ethnic group
- Depression encountered by adoptive parents in the postplacement time period
- The multigenerational challenges faced by aging (kinship) parents as they try to raise their grandchildren

□ Adopted individuals/children/kinship children:
- Attachment issues faced by children/adolescents who have experienced multiple placements and/or lacked consistent care
- Behaviors that are born out of trauma experienced (acute and chronic)
- Physical, emotional, social, and psychological needs of adopted individuals, from placement through the life span.

SUMMARY

After reading this book, the APN will be able to provide safe, quality, informed care that is characterized by best evidence to adoption and kinship triads. Through this care, the social units affected by adoption and kinship practices will be strengthened and those most vulnerable will be optimally served. APNs will become adoption-/kinship-informed caregivers.

CHAPTER HIGHLIGHTS

□ Graduate-level Quality and Safety Education in Nursing (QSEN) as outlined by the American Association of Colleges of Nursing provide six key areas in which practice content related to adoptive and kinship families can be addressed.

□ Quality improvement activities include being an adoption-competent APN.

□ Safe care includes understanding trauma, maltreatment of children, and legal issues.

□ Collaboration with nontraditional team members when caring for families may include adoption agency staff and professionals in the criminal justice system.

□ Patient-centered care is critical for members of these triads and includes withholding judgment as well as a focus on individuals' autonomy and informed consent, and fidelity.

□ APNs' practice is guided by evidence that spans multiple disciplines, an appreciation of the heterogeneity of these groups, and the personal interpretation of the adoption and kinship experience for the individual.

☐ Both adoption practices and policies, as well as APNs' scope of practice, are primarily described and enforced at the state level.

☐ Informatics and access to information are issues within the adoption community. Rights to such information are on the forefront of current conversations. The Internet and social media are drivers in the evolution of such information.

☐ Several nursing organizations' members interface with adoptive and kinship families.

☐ Two major themes are addressed in this guide. Consolidating this information propels the nursing profession forward to deliver quality, patient-centered care. This guide is for both practicing APNs and APN students.

Questions for Reflection

Following are a few questions to reflect upon. You can use these to start a journal for yourself or in a classroom discussion with peers and the instructor.

1. Think of a time in the clinical setting when you were caring for persons who were members of either the adoption or kinship triad. How did you know they were members of these triads? When did you know that they were? Were you comfortable in the delivery of care? What would have made the situation more comfortable for you? For them?

2. Many individuals have strong feelings that are either pro-choice or pro-life. There are also strong feelings about adoption. Some individuals believe that adoptions should not occur and, whenever possible, that birth parents should be given resources to parent their children. Others strongly believe that if parents mistreat their children or are unable to care for them, their parental rights should be terminated in a timely manner. What are your personal views about adoption and kinship care?

References

Adoption Registry Connect. (2015). Worldwide adoptee and birth parent search database. Retrieved from http://adopteeconnect.com/index.htm

American Academy of Pediatrics. (2013). *Helping foster and adoptive families cope with trauma.* Elk Grove Village, IL: American Academy of Pediatrics and Dave Thomas Foundation for Adoption.

American Academy of Pediatrics: Task Force on Healthcare for Children in Foster Care. (2005). *Fostering health: Health care for children and adolescents in foster care* (2nd Ed). Elk Grove Village, IL: American Academy of Pediatrics.

American Adoption Congress. (2016). State legislation. Retrieved from http://www.americanadoptioncongress.org/state.php

American Association of Colleges of Nursing. (2012). *Graduate-level QSEN competencies: Knowledge, skills, and attitudes.* Washington, DC: Author. Retrieved from http://www.aacn.nche.edu/faculty/qsen/competencies .pdf

American College of Obstetricians and Gynecologists. (2012). Adoption: Committee Opinion No. 528. *Obstetrics & Gynecology, 119,* 1320–1324.

American Society of Reproductive Medicine. (2014). Fact sheet/adoption: Where to start and what to think about. Birmingham, AL: Author. Retrieved from http://www.reproductivefacts.org/uploadedFiles/ASRM_Content /Resources/Patient_Resources/Fact_Sheets_and_Info_Booklets/ Adoption-Fact.pdf_

Child Welfare Information Gateway. (2010). Kinship caregivers and the child welfare system. Retrieved from https://www.childwelfare.gov/ pubPDFs/f_kinshi.pdf

Child Welfare Information Gateway. (2011). Searching for birth relatives. Retrieved from https://www.childwelfare.gov/pubPDFs/f_search.pdf

Children's Bureau: U.S. Department of Health and Human Services. (2011). *Child welfare outcomes 2008–2011: Report to Congress.* Retrieved from http://www.acf.hhs.gov/sites/default/files/cb/cwo08_11.pdf

Conn, A. M., Szilagyi, M. A., Franke, T. M., Albertin, C. S., Blumkin, A. K., & Szilagyi, P. G. (2013). Trends in child protection and out-of-home care. *Pediatrics, 132*(4), 712–719. doi:10.1542/peds.2013-0969

Independent Search Consultants. (2001). Retrieved from http://www .iscsearch.com/home.htm

Indiana Department of Health. (2015). Adoption registry. Retrieved from https://adoptiondatabase.quickbase.com/db/7c2gsmqv?a=q&qid=68

International Soundex Reunion Registry. (2011–2012). Changing the world one reunion at a time. Retrieved from http://www.isrr.org

Mason, P., Johnson, D., & Prock, L. A. (2014). *Adoption medicine: Caring for children and families*. Elk Grove Village, IL: American Academy of Pediatrics.

National Council for Adoption. (2014). Federal adoption policy: Privacy in adoption. Retrieved from https://www.adoptioncouncil.org/who-we -are/mission/Federal-Adoption-Policy

National Court Appointed Special Advocates Association. (2015). *The solution: Citizen volunteers*. Retrieved from http://www.casaforchildren .org

Patient Protection and Affordable Care Act, 42 U.S.C. § 18001 (2010).

Pemberton, C. K., Neiderhiser, J. M., Leve, L. D., Natsuaki, M. N., Shaw, D. S., Reiss, D., Ge, X. (2010). Influence of parental depressive symptoms on adopted toddler behaviors: An emerging developmental cascade of genetic and environmental effects. *Developmental Psychopathology, 22,* 803–818. doi: 10.1017/S09545794100004774

Tully, E. C., Iacono, W. G., McGue, M. (2008). An adoption study of parental depression as an environmental liability for adolescent depression and childhood disruptive disorders. *The American Journal of Psychiatry, 165,* 1148–1154.

Vandivere, S., Malm, K., & Radel, L. (2009). *Adoption USA: A chartbook based on the 2007 National Survey of Adoptive Parents*. Washington, DC: The U.S. Department of Health and Human Services, Office of the Assistant Secretary for Planning and Evaluation.

1

Adoption and Kinship Parenting: A Historical, Cultural, and Legal Perspective

□ □ □ □

PURPOSE OF THE CHAPTER

In this chapter, we focus on the historical, cultural, and legal landscape that has shaped adoption and kinship care in the United States. Looking back over the past 150 years, I realize how adoption and kinship parenting are proxies for societal norms contextualized by historical perspectives on class, race, gender, and parental and child rights. It is a fascinating history, and once you examine the waves of change and realize a significant wave of change is happening now, you understand how important it is for advanced practice nurses (APNs) to advocate for those whose lives are impacted. Think of this chapter as "Adoption and Kinship Families: 101" containing important information that lays the foundation for subsequent chapters.

Learning Objectives

At the completion of the chapter, the reader will be able to:

1. Describe historical, cultural, and legal influences of adoption and kinship care in the United States from the late 1800s through today
2. Appreciate the evolution of individual triad's societal positions and rights, which are based in contexts of social mores

3. Describe the types of adoption, trends in adoption (i.e., domestic versus intercountry), and processes involved in adopting a child
4. Become culturally aware of minority groups whose cultural patterns have been marginalized in society (e.g., Native Americans and African Americans)
5. Articulate the influence of the media in presenting adoption in popular culture
6. Form an awareness of the personal attitudes toward adoption, either through direct experiences or via family and friends whose lives have been touched by adoption

ADOPTION IN THE UNITED STATES

Adoption and kinship practices in the United States are entering into a new era of openness, connections (after adoption), and distributions of power that include the birth parents and individuals who are adopted. There is a call to "adopt reform" (The Donaldson Adoption Institute [DAI], 2016) that is compelling in its mission to reframe adoption as a lifelong transformation. Ten areas are outlined by DAI to undertake this transformation:

1. Advocating for standardization of processes, such as the home study
2. Unrestricted access to original birth certificates for adopted individuals
3. Open adoptions and building relationships between birth and adoptive families
4. Increased public support for pre- and postadoption services
5. Explicit state bans on unregulated custody transfers ("rehoming")
6. Clear depiction of adoption in society to avoid stigma and stereotypes
7. Screening of prospective adoptive parents without regard to marital status or sexual orientation
8. Working to unite the adoption community as a whole
9. Removing the influence of money in adoptions, and decreasing the perception of children as commodities
10. Uniform regulations in the use of technology used to connect birth and adoptive families (DAI, 2016)

These are important goals, some with long historical roots, and others, such as unregulated custodies, more recent. To fully understand how this declaration departs from, connects with, and expands upon today's practices, let us start at the beginning.

HISTORY OF ADOPTION IN THE UNITED STATES

An individual does not have to look hard to see examples of adoption throughout history. There is, it would seem, an instinctive aspect to adoption, an intuitive aspect to it. The practice is not just confined to humans, but includes other species that chose to parent the offspring of others. Such parenting may mean life or death to the being adopted. For humans, adoption goes back to ancient times (Conn, 2013). For example, the story of Moses describes a Hebrew woman who seeks protection for her newborn son and sets the infant afloat in a river. The baby is rescued, and ultimately adopted by the pharaoh's daughter and raised as a royal prince. Adoption in the United States has a fluid historical narrative as well as a much more polarized nature. The picture of adoption today is colored by myriad contexts: social, legal, racial, and cultural injustices; misogyny/women's rights/reproduction; religion; and, finally, politics, federal policy, and state statutes. The history of social work in the United States is also threaded in the story of adoption and has influenced the way adoption was manifested throughout the 20th century.

Only fairly recently have there been statistics to help us realize, as a society, the number of individuals involved in adoption and kinship care. The federal system of collecting state information via Title IV-E agencies was established in 1986 and is called the Adoption and Foster Care Analysis and Reporting System (AFCARS). The AFCARS collects data on all children who have been in foster care and/or adopted through services of Title IV-E agencies. Yet we still do not have exact numbers that reflect all adoptions: Private adoptions are often not reported to public databases, and kinship care may be informal, without child welfare agency involvement. It was not until 2000 that the U.S. census even asked questions pertaining to adoption (Conn, 2013). Regardless, adoption is part of our nation's past and as a modern society—it is estimated that 60% of us have some connection to adoption (Pertman, 2000).

Although a retelling of the history of adoption is beyond the purpose of this text, there are watershed moments that need to be described to assist APNs in understanding the patients who stand, sit, and lie before them. Influences overlap, and the telling of this history is not well demarcated in some instances. It is a messy story, with outcomes grounded in the effects of war, religion, women's rights, and the history of family. The 20th and 21st centuries marked the beginning of what we now think of as modern adoption.

THE CREATION OF LEGALIZED ADOPTION

The first landmark in the history of adoption occurred in 1851 when the State of Massachusetts passed "An Act to Provide for the Adoption of Children" (Conn, 2013). Although informal arrangements had been practiced for centuries in America, this law was the first to regulate adoption and was used as a model for other states that quickly passed similar laws (Conn, 2013). Although this was a significant state law, it also symbolized the protection of children who were not born to their parents: the philosophical stronghold of "in the best interest of the child" was born. The law also took into consideration the fitness of the adoptive parents. In sum, it created a new legal family that was overseen by states: an adoptive family. Conn (2013) acknowledges this as a reflection of America's plurality: "In short, America, that nursery of reinvention, would re-invent families as well as individuals" (p. 72).

ORPHAN TRAINS

About this time, in 1853, Charles Loring Brace, a minister, founded the New York Children's Aid Society (Kahan, 2006). The mission of the Children's Aid Society was to save children who were living in poverty and move them away from the institutions that many of these children were forced to live in (orphan asylums and almshouses). Partly because of the influx of immigrants, these urban dwellings for children became places of hunger, crime, and poverty. Brace's idea was to relocate children from the poor environments of the city to rural areas where they could be adopted by welcoming parents

(Kahan, 2006). Recruited from almshouses, places of horrid conditions, the streets, and even families, children were set on trains to all 50 states looking for homes (Conn, 2013). Children were placed on a platform to be examined by prospective parents; thus, the term "put up" for adoption was coined (Kahan, 2006). From 1854 through the 1930s, orphan trains transported children from Eastern cities to be adopted across the country. Approximately 250,000 orphaned or abandoned children were eventually carried to cities across the county (Conn, 2013). Little follow-up was performed to determine whether the orphan trains were indeed placing children in safe conditions. Historical narratives report mixed outcomes for these children.

THE PROGRESSIVE ERA: THE CHILDREN'S BUREAU AND THE CHILD WELFARE LEAGUE OF AMERICA

As all wars do, the Civil War created widows and orphans. The first orphanages were seen during the post-Civil War time, and they continued to grow (Conn, 2013). In 1909, the White House Conference on the Care of Dependent Children was convened to discuss the 93,000 children living in orphanages and the 50,000 in foster care (Kahan, 2006). Several factors are of note during the progressive era: (a) the ideological shift toward family preservation surfaced, including the passage of Mother's Pensions, aimed at covering the costs of raising children; (b) social work as a profession to oversee adoption practices took hold; and (c) governmental responsibility in overseeing adoption practices was initiated (Conn, 2013; Kahan, 2006). In the mid-1930s, children living in orphanages rose sharply to nearly 150,000 children; however, by the end of the decade, these numbers began to decrease as legal adoptions rose (Conn, 2013). Indeed, adoptions tripled between 1937 and 1945, and then doubled in 1955 (Kahan, 2006).

The first federal agency to act on behalf of children was the Children's Bureau, established in 1912 (Children's Bureau, 2015; see also Children's Bureau Timeline at cb100.acf.hhs.gov/childrens -bureau-timeline). Today, the Children's Bureau, an Office of the Administration for Children and Families, devotes resources to preventing child abuse and neglect, and supporting foster care and adoption services. Although focused on children in the welfare system, the Children's Bureau, through the Child Welfare Information Gateway, has published numerous documents on topics that pertain to adoptive and kinship triads. The information is straightforward and offers helpful answers to a broad array of questions that APNs might have, ranging from health care consent to treat children who are not living with birth parents to reuniting adopted persons with birth parents.

In the private sector, the Child Welfare League of America, the oldest national child-welfare organization, was formed in 1920 (www .cwla.org). This membership-based organization's primary objective is to "make children, especially our most vulnerable children, a priority in the United States" (Child Welfare League of America, 2013). Today, the Child Welfare League sponsors conferences, disseminates new policy information, and provides training and consulting services.

WORLD WAR II, THE KOREAN CONFLICT, AND INTERNATIONAL ADOPTION

As we have learned, wars create orphans and single parent situations, which in turn create the need for domestic adoptions. Wars also create orphans in other countries. Two surges in adoption came in the aftermath of World War II and the Korean Conflict (1950–1953), both of which left thousands of children without parents and homes. During the mid-1940s, intercountry adoption began in America (Brumble & Kampfe, 2011). European orphans after World War II primarily came from Germany and Greece (Brumble & Kampfe, 2011). Adoptions from Korea also marked the beginning of transracial adoptions—for the first time in American history; children were being adopted by parents of a different race. One couple, Harry and Bertha Holt, adopted eight Korean children, advocated for a change in federal law to do so, and started Holt International, one of the largest international adoption agencies today (Brumble & Kampfe, 2011). Other adoption agencies that included and specialized in intercountry adoption grew, and this growth continued through the 1960s. Part of this surge was attributed to the Civil Rights movement and new-founded tolerance to differences (Brumble & Kampfe, 2011). The geopolitical ramifications of adoption became more salient as children were transported outside of their countries of origin.

Special needs adoptions came into being at this time as well. Given that the federal government does not have an accepted definition of special needs, identification of special needs within the context of domestic and intercountry adoptions may differ. Qualifying for adoption assistance by the federal or state governments, however, requires that children meet certain eligibility requirements. A straightforward definition is presented by Brumble and Kampfe (2011): "Special needs adoption is the adoption of children who are older, bi-racial, had to be placed with their siblings, or had mental, physical, or emotional problems" (p. 159). Therefore, a child may be physically healthy, but still be labeled as "special needs."

THE BABY SCOOP ERA: 1945 TO 1972

In addition to the growth of intercountry adoption and the practice of special needs adoption, domestic-born infants became more in demand in the 1960s. This demand created concerns about the treatment of birth mothers. The Child Welfare League of America (1960) published its *Standards for Services to Unmarried Parents*, and in Chapter 2: Reaching Out to Unmarried Mothers (Child Welfare League of America, 1960), it issued ethical cautions regarding this demand for infants:

> Because of the current widespread demand for adoptable white children, there are many people in the community who are ready to offer assistance to the unmarried mother, either for personal gain or to secure the child for themselves or for other interested persons. Intervention of such people, even when they are well-meaning, presents hazards to many children, unmarried mothers, and adoptive families. In accepting such help, the unmarried mother may make plans for the child which are not in accordance with her basic wishes, or [the child's] best interest, and may be deprived of professional services concerned with her own welfare and future adjustment. (p. 11)

The document also specifically states that unwed pregnancy should not be "made a reason for referral to state training schools for girls or to the state reformatory" (p. 12). There is mention of vocational counseling and other services to support the mother and child. Nurses are specifically cited several times as one of the first points of contact for the unwed mother. The historical text is clear, however, that the needs of the child are paramount. What is also clear is that the caseworker/social worker is the professional who is charged with teasing out these needs (Child Welfare League, 1960). The document further clarifies that when "helping" the mother in deciding whether to keep the child "[s]ocial sanctions militate against a mother's bringing up an out-of-wedlock child" (p. 19).

The discourse reveals a sense of altruism in wanting to help the mother and child within the context of mores and norms of the time. This humanity toward and support of the birth mother is juxtaposed with the practices of closed adoptions by strangers and a psychoanalytic model of single mothers as espoused by social workers (Baby Scoop Era, n.d.). The Baby Scoop Era in American history signifies the thirst for children in post–World War II society and, some would argue, the use of coercion and shame placed upon birth mothers to place their children for adoption (Baby Scoop Era, n.d.). During this phase, matching of physical characteristics was not uncommon.

LEGALIZATION OF ABORTION, AVAILABILITY OF CONTRACEPTION, AND DECREASED STIGMA TO UNWED PREGNANCIES

However, other movements were also changing the societal landscape and, therefore, adoption practices. Social mores changed significantly in the mid- to late 1960s with the onset of liberalized, open-minded thinking, and the Great Society, including the creation of government health care programs such as Medicare and Medicaid. Not only did the 1960s and 1970s herald new civil rights, trends in relinquishments also shifted after the legalization of abortion in the case of *Roe vs. Wade* in 1973, and availability of contraception (e.g., "the Pill"; Kahan, 2006). This watershed federal law and the reproductive technology of oral contraceptives offered women newfound choices regarding motherhood. The result was a dramatic decrease in the number of available infants and children for adoption and a renewed interest in intercountry adoption (Brumble & Kampfe, 2011).

Adoptive parents continued to seek infants through special needs and transracial adoptions. Record numbers of minority children, often African American, were placed with White parents. Social workers "aggressively recruited adoptive families for African American children," which peaked in 1971 (Kahan, 2006). Influenced by the trends in the 1960s and the era of Black pride, as well as the number of children placed with White families, in 1972, the National Association of Black Social Workers (NABSW) issued a "Position Statement on Trans-Racial Adoptions":

> The National Association of Black Social Workers has taken vehement stand against the placement of Black children in white homes for any reason. . . . (p. 1)
>
> Special programming in learning to handle Black children's hair, learning Black culture, "trying to become Black", puts normal family activities in the form of special family projects to accommodate the odd member of the family. . . . (p. 2)

As a result of this position statement, transracial adoptions fell by 39% that year (Kahan, 2006). Today, transracial adoptions—domestic and intercountry—continue to have both advocates and individuals who argue passionately against such practice.

By the 1980s, open adoptions, search narratives, and birth mothers' efforts to find their children also entered into the cultural landscape and society's conversations surrounding adoption (Kahan, 2006; Melosh, 2002). Interestingly, nurse scholars identified the long-term effects on birth mothers of relinquishing a child. Askren and Bloom (1999) performed a systematic literature review, with 12 articles spanning the years 1978 to 1994, and concluded that the birth mother's grief reaction was unique and lifelong. This grief placed her at risk for physical, psychological, and social "repercussions" (p. 395). The authors also concluded that the mother was susceptible to chronic, unresolved grief (Askren & Bloom, 1999).

In the 1990s with the decline of communism, the entry of the United States into a global economy reignited the trend of U.S. parents seeking children from other countries who may also be classified as special needs (Brumble & Kampfe, 2011). During this time, many children from the former Soviet Union were adopted into the United

States. The effects of sensory deprivation, inconsistent caregiving/ meeting of the child's needs, neglect, and longer exposure to adverse conditions were evident in these children who had been cared for in Soviet orphanages and brought to the United States (Brumble & Kampfe, 2011). Many of these children manifested extraordinary medical, developmental, and behavioral needs, which adoptive parents were unprepared to address. Recent declines in the availability of infants from developing countries and the Hague Convention on the Protection of Children and Co-operation in Respect of Intercountry Adoption (Hague Convention) have resulted in a great decrease in the number of children adopted from other countries (see the sections that follow).

Most recently, the United States has recognized the significant need for permanent placements of children in the foster care system. Two federal laws, the Adoption Assistance and Child Welfare Act of 1980 and the Adoption and Safe Families Act of 1997, support the adoption of children waiting in foster care through subsidies and other guidelines. Both of these acts by the federal government were ideological shifts away from reunification of children with their birth families and toward support of adoption and permanent placements (Kahan, 2006). Although social work is still considered the profession that oversees placement of children, other disciplines have emerged to enter into the conversations surrounding the child, including psychology and members of the health care team.

HEGEMONIC FORCES IN ADOPTION AND THOSE WHO NOW SPEAK

Hegemony, as defined by the *Merriam-Webster Dictionary*, is: "1: preponderant influence or authority over others: domination; 2: the social, cultural, ideological, or economic influence exerted by a dominant group" (Hegemony, 2016). In critical theory and through an examination of discourse, we understand that such hegemony has influenced both domestic and intercountry adoptions. Let us discuss adopted individuals first, and look at how some are embracing a unique discourse.

Adopted persons have asserted an opposing narrative, one in objection to amended and sealed birth certificates. The most well-known alternative discourse is voiced by members of the group Bastard

---

EXHIBIT 1.1
BASTARD NATION MISSION STATEMENT

Bastard Nation is dedicated to the recognition of the full human and civil rights of adult adoptees. Toward that end, we advocate the opening to adoptees, upon request at age of majority, of those government documents which pertain to the adoptee's historical, genetic, and legal identity, including the unaltered original birth certificate and adoption decree. Bastard Nation asserts that it is the right of people everywhere to have their official original birth records unaltered and free from falsification, and that the adoptive status of any person should not prohibit him or her from choosing to exercise that right. We have reclaimed the badge of bastardy placed on us by those who would attempt to shame us; we see nothing shameful in having been born out of wedlock or in being adopted. Bastard Nation does not support mandated mutual consent registries or intermediary systems in place of unconditional open records, nor any other system that is less than access on demand to the adult adoptee, without condition, and without qualification.

Source: Bastard Nation (2016).

Nation (2016). Their mission statement advocates for political action, but there is more than that in their language (Exhibit 1.1). Words used by the individuals of Bastard Nation reflect individual rights, embracing language that defies shame and stigma and demanding policy changes. This alternate view of adopted persons' rights to full disclosure juxtaposes the charter "in the best interest of the child," as those who decide "best interest" often have not consulted those most affected.

Birth mothers have found their voices as well, some of whom have published accounts of relinquishment, search narratives, and reunions (Melosh, 2002). Search "narratives" as a genre surrounding adoption began in the 1970s and challenged the notion that once children were placed, their story ended (Melosh, 2002). In the 1980s and 1990s, these narratives increased in number, were read by broader audiences, and took on the arc of a search and reunion story (Melosh, 2002, p. 245). Issues related to identity, informed consent, secrecy of being adopted, and birth family reunions upended long-held assumptions about the practices of adoption and less powerful members of the adoption triad. Conversations about these topics continue today.

ADOPTION LAW

Adoption's history over the past 150 years has translated into the laws that govern its practices. As mentioned earlier, how adoption is practiced is primarily dictated by state statutes with significant federal constitutional and statutory laws. Although there are variations across states, characteristics of today's modern adoption laws specify (a) complete transfer of parental rights to the adoptive parents; (b) requirement of birth parent(s) consent; (c) the best interest of the child as a guiding standard; (d) the confidential nature of the adoption proceedings; and (e) the permanency of the adoption (Acosta, 2013). Let us briefly discuss these characteristics.

In addition to parental rights being transferred to the adoptive parent, the responsibilities of parentage are also conferred. For example, the adopted child has the same rights as biological offspring, including inheritance and tax laws. The transfer of rights to the adoptive parents is simultaneous with the termination of parental rights (Acosta, 2013). In the case of voluntary termination, full consent by the biological mother is required in all 50 states. Consent of married fathers is also usually required. In the cases of unmarried fathers, many states have registries for putative (presumed or alleged) fathers to voluntarily offer contact information so that notification of adoption proceedings may occur. Federal law also stipulates that if the father demonstrates a substantial interest in the child, his right to consent must be honored. The best interest of the child has been interpreted to mean that these interests come before biological or adoptive parent rights. Postplacement visits during a probationary period are made to adoptive homes to ensure that the child's interests are being supported. Adoption proceedings are confidential:

> The records of the adoption proceeding are sealed and may not be opened except upon a judicial finding of good cause,

or in some states upon the mutual consent of all parties. The child's original birth certificate is sealed, and a new one is issued containing only the child's adoptive name. (Acosta, 2013)

Adoptions are also considered permanent, after a state's waiting period. This creates a bond between the child and the adoptive parent that is not subject to revocation (Acosta, 2013).

Influences of federal laws are also of note (see Figure 1.1). The first is Constitutional law: the 14th Amendment, Due Process Clause, which gives "natural" (a term contested by many in the adoption

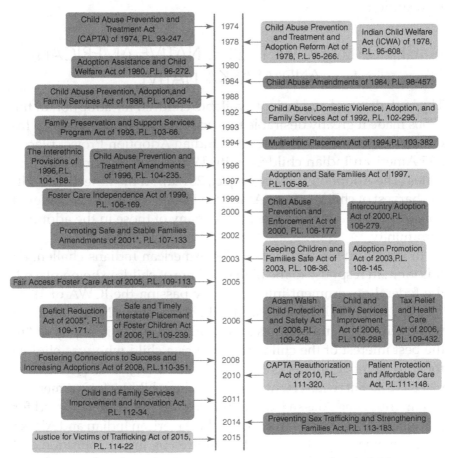

FIGURE 1.1   *Timeline of major federal legislation concerned with child protection, child welfare, and adoption.*

Source: Child Welfare Information Gateway (2016b).

community) parents the liberty to raise and manage their children. Within the context of adoption, this law pertains to termination of parental rights, which rests on "clear and convincing evidence" (Acosta, 2013). Preponderance of evidence findings is insufficient in these cases. The second type of federal law that influences adoption practices are federal statutory laws that support, promote, and at times, regulate state laws. An example would be the Adoption and Safe Families Act of 1997, which promotes state programs that encourage the adoption of children in foster care (Acosta, 2013). The Indian Child Welfare Act (ICWA) of 1978 serves as a federal mandate pertaining to children adopted from tribes, which is described in the next section.

CHILDREN FROM TRIBES: NATIVE AMERICAN AND ALASKA NATIVE

The high demand and lack of available children for adoption in the 1950s made it greatly desirable to place children from American Indian tribes. From 1958 to 1967, the Indian Adoption Project placed 395 American Indian children with White families across several states (The Adoption History Project, 2012a). At the time, the resulting harvest of children from American Indian tribes was considered an enlightened adoption practice by many of those in the adoption community.

In the late 1960s and early 1970s, American Indians challenged this view. In response to the high numbers of children being placed, the federal government intervened by passing the ICWA of 1978. This Act sought to keep American Indian and Alaska Native children with their tribes and families and supported the philosophy of "in the best interest of the child" (defined as a child who was eligible for or a member of a federally recognized tribe). This federal law placed stringent requirements on states when children from American Indian tribes and Alaska Native children were being considered for placement. This federal law protects the American Indian and Alaska Native biological parental rights conferred by the Constitution and effectively reversed the Indian Adoption Project. The law is also of note because, unlike the American doctrine of individualism, the ICWA advocated for tribal rights (The Adoption History Project, 2012b).

In 1983, the Northwest Indian Child Welfare Institute was created, and it later evolved into the National Indian Child Welfare Association (NICWA, 2015; www.nicwa.org). The NICWA is a private, nonprofit organization designed to advocate for American Indian children and prevent child abuse and neglect within the tribal capacity.

ADOPTION TODAY

In addition to social work, other disciplines, such as nursing, psychology, human development, and pediatric medicine, are paying attention to members of the adoption triad. Research continues to be weighted on the principle of the best interest of the child, which is interpreted as child outcomes. Discussions of postadoption services also revolve around the child and needed services. Today, most adoptive families fare well and demonstrate resiliency through an ability to adapt to stressors. In an integrative review of 38 empirical studies on adoptive families published between 1985 and 2003, O'Brien and Zamostny (2003) concluded that adoptive families generally reported satisfaction with "the adoption, family functioning, and parent/child communication" (p. 690). However, it was also noted that many studies had methodological weaknesses and tended to be descriptive. There was a call for additional theory-driven and methodologically sound outcomes research (O'Brien & Zamostny, 2003). In each of the following chapters, we review literature findings pertinent to these triads. Without such conscious knowledge-building, APNs' frames of reference with adoptive and kinship families may stem from personal experiences only and, therefore, be limited. In contrast, with knowledge of the full context of adoption and kinship families, APNs can assess, manage, and treat health conditions with which families present.

TYPES OF ADOPTION IN THE UNITED STATES

In the United States, there are three major paths or types of adoptions: foster care adoption (i.e., child welfare or domestic public adoption); private domestic adoption; and intercountry or international adoption (Vandivere, Malm, & Radel, 2009). The first type of adoption, foster care adoption, occurs when a child is placed with one or two

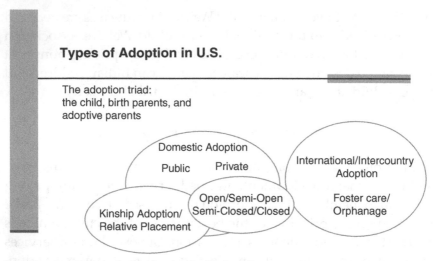

Types of Adoption in U.S.

The adoption triad:
the child, birth parents, and
adoptive parents

Domestic Adoption

Public   Private

International/Intercountry
Adoption

Open/Semi-Open
Semi-Closed/Closed

Foster care/
Orphanage

Kinship Adoption/
Relative Placement

FIGURE 1.2   *Types of adoption in the United States.*

adoptive parents from the child welfare system after being removed from the parents' home because of an inability or unwillingness of the birth parents to care for the child. These types of adoption account for 37% (661,000) of all adoptions in the United States (Vandivere et al., 2009) and, because of recent laws, are increasing (see Figure 1.2).

The Fostering Connections to Success and Increasing Adoptions Act of 2008, signed into law by President George W. Bush, signaled changes to the child welfare system, primarily to Title IV-E of the Social Security Act. Title IV-E covers federal payments to states for foster care and adoption assistance. Of note with this historic law were provisions to keep sibling groups together and to allow states the option to provide kinship guardianship payments or payments to relative foster parents. In 2011, foster care provided by a relative jumped to 29% (of all foster care placements) in the United States (Child Welfare Information Gateway, 2016a). This figure does not include kinship parents who are not officially accessing the foster care/child welfare system.

Not all children in the foster care system are eligible for adoption because issues of termination of parental rights and age of the child (over 16 and waiting for emancipation) play a role. In 2014, a total of 415,000 children were in foster care, an increase from 401,000 in 2013, with 108,000 children waiting to be adopted (U.S. Department of Health and Human Services [DHHS], 2015). The number of children who were adopted remained stable over the past decade (i.e., 50,000 to 52,000; DHHS, 2015).

Multiple cultural connotations—often negative—have surrounded foster care adoptions. Because families see these children as high risk with special needs, many of these children are discounted as potential family members. To promote adoption from the foster care system, AdoptUSKids (www.adoptuskids.org), a project of the U.S. Children's Bureau, was created and provides the only federally funded photo listing of children and youth. AdoptUSKids works with the National Resource Center for Diligent Recruitment (NRCDR), which provides "technical assistance, tools, coaching, and other support to help states, tribes, and territories create lasting systemic changes to improve safety, permanency, and well-being outcomes for children, youth, and families" (National Resource Center for Diligent Recruitment, 2016).

Private domestic adoptions account for 38% of all adoptions (677,000 children; Vandivere et al., 2009) and are arranged between prospective parents and adoption agencies, facilitators, and attorneys. Independent adoptions may be arranged without the use of licensed adoption agencies; instead, prospective parents use adoption facilitators or attorneys. These children are not part of the foster care system and are often infants when they are adopted.

Social media is impacting the way private adoptions are negotiated. Long waits have characterized private adoptions, and increasingly, prospective parents are creating their own Internet messages via social media, such as Facebook and personal websites. Popular culture has called these "DIY adoptions," or Do It Yourself adoptions. Websites such as America Adopts! (www.americaadopts.com) hosts a virtual meeting place for both prospective and expectant parents to connect, designed to supplement the use of adoption agencies and attorneys. Such sites claim that birth parents, who may not be ready to approach an agency, feel more comfortable and in control by reading profiles online. Individuals who use virtual DIY adoption mechanisms should be advised that they may be vulnerable to scams, and to work with a licensed adoption agency. Many individuals will post toll-free numbers, withhold their last names, and use additional protective methods to lessen the risks of being taken advantage of.

Intercountry or internationally adopted children account for 25% of adoptions (444,000 children; Vandivere et al., 2009) and were born outside of the United States. The United States, France, and Spain have the highest numbers of intercountry adoptions (United Nations, Department of Economic and Social Affairs, 2009). These countries are called "receiving countries." In contrast, the major "sending countries," which account for over half of children who are adopted from abroad, are China, Guatemala, the Republic of Korea, the Russian Federation, and the Ukraine (United Nations, Department of Economic and Social Affairs, 2009).

Intercountry adoptions have undergone dramatic shifts because the Hague Convention on the Protection of Children and Co-operation in Respect of Intercountry Adoption (Hague Convention) entered into force in the United States in 2008. This treaty grew from the increased intercountry adoptions seen in the 1960s and 1970s and the concerns over child trafficking (United Nations, Department of Economic and Social Affairs, 2009). A "central authority" is designated by countries that have ratified the treaty (Rotabi & Gibbons, 2012). Select sending countries also began to limit or suspend intercountry adoptions and include the Republic of Korea, Romania, Vietnam, and Uruguay (United Nations, Department of Economic and Social Affairs, 2009). Some countries allow international adoptions to occur only when all efforts to adopt within the country have been exhausted, which reputable adoption agencies strive to do by supporting foster care and domestic adoption programs (S. Horton-Bobo, personal communication, June 14, 2016).

International adoptions have decreased in many countries. For example, China, an approved Hague Convention adoption partner, sent 2,696 children in 2012, 2,306 children in 2013, and 2,040 children in 2014 to the United States to be adopted (U.S. Department of State, Bureau of Consular Affairs, 2015). Table 1.1 depicts the decrease in the number of infants and children adopted in the United States from sending countries from 2004 to 2014. To offset these trends, adoptive parents and agencies have received children from "new" countries, such as Ethiopia.

Although small in number, it should be noted that the United States is also a sending country, whose children, including African American, can be adopted by parents in European countries such

TABLE 1.1　*Number of Intercountry Children Received 2004 to 2014*

United States	
Year	Number of Intercountry Children Received
2004	22,884
2005	22,739
2006	20,679
2007	19,613
2008	17,438
2009	12,753
2010	12,149
2011	9,320
2012	8,668
2013	7,094
2014	6,441
2004–2014	159,778

Adapted from Selman (2015).

as the Netherlands (Brown, 2013). In 2014, 96 U.S. children were adopted to various countries around the world (U.S. Department of State, Bureau of Consular Affairs, 2015).

Multiple national adoption organizations work to support, facilitate, and enhance understanding of adoption in the United States (see Table 1.2). Some have long histories of fulfilling their missions (e.g., Children's Bureau) and others have been formed more recently (e.g., The National Center on Adoption and Permanency). Organizations also may have a domestic adoption focus (e.g., the National Council on Adoptable Children), whereas others are directed toward ensuring the ethical standards in intercountry adoption (e.g., the Joint Council on International Children's Services). APNs will find Table 1.2 helpful as they learn more about the organized efforts to support adoption.

As can be discerned from the history of adoption, the practices in the United States have swung between the commodification of children without regard for birth family rights, to attempts to preserve the original family unit, to finding a balance that lies in the interest of the person at the center: the child. Interpretation of the tenet "in the best interest of the child" has often been fluid and dependent on the social, cultural, and legal standards of the time.

TABLE 1.2 *Major Adoption Organizations in the United States*

Name/Address/Website	Mission/Description
AdoptUSKids 605 Global Way, Suite 100 Linthicum, MD 21090 adoptuskids.org	AdoptUSKids' mission: (1) To raise public awareness about the need for foster and adoptive families for children in the public child welfare system; and (2) to assist U.S. states, territories, and tribes to recruit and retain foster and adoptive families.
American Academy of Adoption Attorneys P.O. Box 33053 Washington, DC 20033 www.adoptionattorneys.org/	The American Academy of Adoption Attorneys is a national association of approximately 340 attorneys who practice, or have otherwise distinguished themselves, in the field of adoption law. The Academy's work includes promoting the reform of adoption laws and disseminating information on ethical adoption practices.
Center for Adoption Support and Education (C.A.S.E.) 4000 Blackburn Lane, Suite 260 Burtonsville, MD 20866 adoptionsupport.org	The Center for Adoption Support and Education (C.A.S.E.) strengthens the well-being of foster and adoptive families, promotes adoption awareness, enhances adoption sensitivity, and develops the skills for professionals and families to empower children to thrive.
Child Welfare Information Gateway Children's Bureau/ACYF 1250 Maryland Avenue SW, Eighth FloorWashington, DC 20024 www.childwelfare.gov/topics/preventing/promoting/parenting/relative/	Connecting child welfare and related professionals to comprehensive resources to help protect children and strengthen families.
Congressional Coalition on Adoption Institute 311 Massachusetts Avenue NE Washington, DC 20002 www.ccainstitute.org	The Congressional Coalition on Adoption Institute is dedicated to raising awareness about the millions of children around the world in need of permanent, safe, and loving families and to eliminating the barriers that hinder these children from realizing their basic right to a family.

The Dave Thomas Foundation for Adoption is driven by a single goal: finding a loving family for every child waiting in foster care to get adopted. We are America's only national nonprofit charity dedicated solely to finding permanent homes for the more than 100,000 children in foster care.

The Donaldson Adoption Institute's mission is to better the lives of everyone touched by adoption through sound research, education and advocacy that improves laws, policies and practices.

The JCICS advances the overall well-being of vulnerable children and their right to live in permanent family care. This organization brings its mission to life through programs and services designed to ensure children live in safe, permanent, strong families.

Passionately committed to the belief that every child deserves to thrive in a nurturing, permanent family, NCFA's mission is to meet the diverse needs of children, birthparents, adopted individuals, adoptive families, and all those touched by adoption through global advocacy, education, research, legislative action, and collaboration.

NACAC promotes and supports permanent families for children and youth in the United States and Canada—especially children and youth who are or have been in foster care and those with special needs.

Dave Thomas Foundation for Adoption
716 Mt. Airyshire Blvd., Suite 100
Columbus, OH 43235
davethomasfoundation.org

The Donaldson Adoption Institute
120 East 38th Street
New York, NY 10016
adoptioninstitute.org

Joint Council on International Children's Services
117 South Saint Asaph Street
Alexandria, VA 22314
jointcouncil.org

National Council for Adoption
225 N. Washington Street
Alexandria, VA 22314
adoptioncouncil.org

North American Council on Adoptable Children
970 Raymond Avenue, Suite 106
St. Paul, MN 55114
nacac.org

(continued)

TABLE 1.2 *Major Adoption Organizations in the United States (continued)*

Name/Address/Website	Mission/Description
National Center on Adoption and Permanency Contact: Adam Pertman, President at apertman@ncap-us.org nationalcenteronadoptionandpermanency.net	The National Center for Adoption and Permanency (NCAP) is a unique "one-stop" national organization that provides a broad range of multidisciplinary services and resources relating to adoption, foster care and child welfare. The consultancy—through its website and its team of highly experienced and successful trainers, educators, speakers, and presenters—is designed to provide a single destination where agencies, government entities at all levels, conference organizers, family and advocacy groups, and professionals can go for expert services and consulting, reliable information, and other assistance to fill their short-term and strategic needs.
U.S. Department of State, Bureau of Consular Affairs, Office of Children's Issues. CA/OCS/CI SA-17, 9th Floor Washington, DC 20522-1709 adoption.state.gov	The Office of Children's Issues (CI), part of the Bureau of Consular Affairs at the U.S. Department of State, plays an active role in the intercountry adoption process. In our work, we are dedicated to assisting parents as they seek to provide a home to orphans abroad. The Bureau of Consular Affairs carries out the Department of State's responsibilities as the U.S. Central Authority for the Hague Adoption Convention. The Office of Children's Issues is responsible for the day-to-day oversight and implementation of the Hague Adoption Convention in the United States.

POPULAR CULTURE AND THE POLITICAL CONTEXT OF ADOPTIVE FAMILIES

Just as there is an intersection between loss and healing in adoption and kinship families, so, too, there is a contrast in how popular culture and society view these families. In one perspective, there is a sense that adoption is for the "rich and famous" and, simultaneously, for parents who cannot have their "own" children through birth. Viewed by many as a practice for the elite, adoption is still considered by some to be a second-best alternative to building a family. Several celebrities have opted to become single adoptive parents: Sandra Bullock, Diane Keaton, Meg Ryan, and Charlize Theron. Others, such as Madonna and Guy Ritchie, Tom Cruise and Nicole Kidman, and Brad and Angelina Jolie Pitt, and the late Bob Hope have built families with their partners through adoption. Rosie O'Donnell is one of several same-sex parents to build a family through adoption. Several others, including Elton John and Neil Patrick Harris, have children via in vitro fertilization and surrogacy.

Then there are celebrities who are adopted themselves: Former President Bill Clinton, Jesse Jackson, Faith Hill, the late Art Linkletter, and Daunte Culpepper (football player). Famous birth parents include Rosanne Barr, Joni Mitchell, Kate Mulgrew, and David Crosby. Although certainly not an exhaustive list, the nation seems to be obsessed when a person is identified as part of an adoption triad. Often media stories that involve an adoptive family member will be identified, in some cases, without rationale.

KINSHIP FAMILIES

The history of kinship intertwines with that of adoption; however, there are points of departure. First, kinship care was practiced informally before and after the historic 1851 passage of legal adoption in Massachusetts (Conn, 2013). Kinship parents may be adoptive parents (see Figure 1.2), foster parents, guardians, or in an informal arrangement within the family. Second, kinship care has been and is a specific part of African American communities' history and current-day family practices. The National Association of Black Social Workers (2003) prepared a position statement on kinship caregiving:

Informal adoption or the rearing of children by relatives is one of the most enduring African traditions that survived the Middle Passage. During slavery, elderly relatives often reared thousands of children whose parents had been sold as chattel. Informal adoption continues to be widespread in the black community. Today, over two million African American children are raised by grandparents, aunts or uncles, brothers and sisters, cousins and others who are not formal relatives. (p. 2)

Today, one in five Black children will spend time under the care of kinship parents at some point (Annie E. Casey Foundation, 2012). Approximately 31% of Black children live in public or private kinship care, as compared with 40% of White (non-Hispanic) children, and 23% of Hispanic children (Annie E. Casey Foundation, 2012).

The evolution of the name "kinship care" is of note. In 1990, the Child Welfare League of America convened a session of the National Commission on Family Foster Care to discuss the term "foster family care," which was the long-held name for relative foster care (Pasztor, 2015, p.23). Suggestions during this meeting included the revision "family foster care" to indicate the emphasis on family (p. 23). Recalling the book by Carol Stack, *All Our Kin: Strategies for Survival in a Black Community* (1983), Eileen Mayers Pasztor recommended the term "kinship care" (p. 24). Later, Pasztor became the first national program leader for kinship care for the Child Welfare League of America (Pasztor, 2015).

There are several reasons kinship families exist. Incarceration, death, substance abuse, military deployments, maltreatment of a child (neglect and abuse), and other circumstances prevent birth parents from continuing to parent their children. Unlike adoption, there is a relative, close family member, or fictive kin to step in and parent the child. As with many issues related to adoption, states define kinship families/care in different ways. Some states use the criterion of "blood relation" to indicate "relative care" and "kinship care" to indicate non–blood-related individuals, such as godparents, close family friends, teachers, and so forth.

"Fictive kin" is another term used in relation to kinship caregivers, and typically refers to individuals who serve as family members without ties of blood or law (Brathwaite et al., 2010). After reviewing

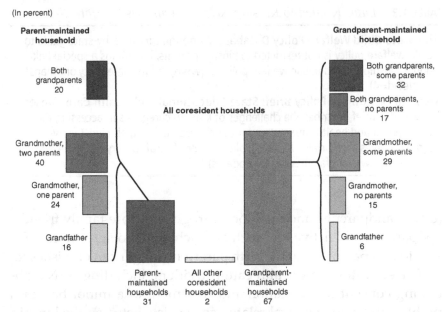

(In percent)

Parent-maintained household

Both grandparents 20

All coresident households

Grandmother, two parents 40

Grandmother, one parent 24

Grandfather 16

Parent-maintained households 31

All other coresident households 2

Grandparent-maintained households 67

Grandparent-maintained household

Both grandparents, some parents 32

Both grandparents, no parents 17

Grandmother, some parents 29

Grandmother, no parents 15

Grandfather 6

FIGURE 1.3   *Households with coresident grandparents and grandchildren.*
Source: Ellis and Simmons (2014).

600 articles with the term "fictive kin," Nelson (2014) asserts that this nomenclature is used more often in relation to African Americans and marginalized groups (gays and lesbians) than Whites and mainstream groups (heterosexual). In contrast, Nelson (2014) inserts new discourse to include "families of choice" and "voluntary kin" (p. 218). Figure 1.3 outlines the various kinship arrangements (Ellis & Simmons, 2014). Sixty-seven percent of these co-resident households are grandparent maintained, indicating that in households with grandparents in residence, most are headed by these individuals.

Health Care and Educational Consent for Children in Kinship Care

The federal government allows states to define what is meant by "relative," and this term in some states includes nonblood kinship caregivers. These definitions are important as they influence who may be eligible for resources. The State Child Welfare Policy Database offers a state-by-state definition of how kin is defined (see Table 1.3). For the purposes of this text, kinship is defined broadly, to include blood

TABLE 1.3   *Laws Related to Kinship/Relative Families by State*

The State Child Welfare Policy Database: Although this state-by-state guide to child welfare policy is not restricted to kinship parents, it contains a special link about kinship-related public welfare policies. (www.childwelfarepolicy.org/maps/single?id=4)

Generations United Policy Brief: State Educational and Health Care Consent Laws: This brief describes the challenges of kinship caregivers in accessing the educational and health care system for the children under their care. (www.grandfamilies.org/Portals/0/GU%20Policy%20Brief%20February%202014.pdf; see also www.grandfamilies.org for updates)

(e.g., grandparents) and nonblood caregivers (close family friends, godparents, and fictive kin, such as teachers) who agree to care for a child as a parent when the birth parent no longer can or wishes to.

For educators and health care providers, including APNs, obtaining consent for education and treatment of a minor becomes problematic when no legal relationship exists between the kinship parent and the child. Typically, to establish such a relationship means legal proceedings that can be emotionally and financially difficult for kinship parents. Power of attorney forms may be challenging to obtain when birth parents refuse to sign papers or cannot be located. Education laws have historically been drafted to protect schools from the parental practice of sending children outside of districts to preferred schools. Documentation of residence is required for public school enrollments; however, kinship parents, who may reside in a district other than the child's, are penalized if they cannot provide evidence of legal custody or guardianship. Similarly, health care laws require a legal relationship to deliver care to avoid litigation and violations of health privacy laws.

In response to these barriers to education and health care, states have passed consent laws whereby kinship parents complete an affidavit, an attestation of the fact that they are the child's caregivers. Currently, no state requires a (birth) parent signature on these forms. Select states place the affidavit form within the consent laws. Despite consent laws, which protect health care workers from liability related to using the affidavit, insurance providers vary with regard to whom they will cover because definitions of "dependent" vary by insurance carriers (see Table 1.3). As of 2013, 15 states have passed educational consent laws, and 24 states have passed health care consent laws (Beltran, 2013).

Kinship Organizations and Resources

I have seen firsthand how kinship families' legal arrangements overlap with adoptive and foster parents. In kinship parenting classes that I cofacilitate, I have had individuals who were kinship parents as well as adoptive parents; kinship parents who were also foster parents; kinship parents who were guardians to the child(ren); and kinships parents who were "off the grid," with no legal arrangement or child welfare involvement with the child(ren). One parent half-jokingly commented, "I'm not legal," when asked what arrangement she had as caregiver to her grandchildren. Similarly, kinship parents' arrangements with the birth parents ranged from supervised visits with the birth parents, to birth parents' transient presence in the home, to coresident households. Table 1.4 outlines several organizations that are specific to kinship parents; but APNs should note that, depending upon the arrangement and legal permanency of the kinship parent, resources listed in Table 1.2 may also be beneficial to kinship caregivers.

TABLE 1.4 *Kinship Parent Organizations/Resources*

Kinship Parent Organizations/Resources	Mission Statements
AARP This website has a multitude of fact sheets and resources for grandparents who are raising grandchildren, including online support groups. AARP 601 E Street NW Washington, DC 20049 www.aarp.org	AARP enhances the quality of life for all as we age. The AARP champions positive social change and deliver value through advocacy, information, and service.
Administration on Aging (AoA) Administration for Community Living 330 C St SW Washington, DC 20201 www.aoa.gov/	The AoA maximizes the independence, well-being, and health of older adults, people with disabilities, and their families and caregivers.

(continued)

TABLE 1.4   *Kinship Parent Organizations/Resources (continued)*

Kinship Parent Organizations/Resources	Mission Statements
Child Welfare Information Gateway Children's Bureau/ACYF 1250 Maryland Avenue SW Eighth Floor Washington, DC 20024 www.childwelfare.gov/topics/preventing/ promoting/parenting/relative/	The Children's Bureau connects child welfare and related professionals to comprehensive resources to help protect children and strengthen families.
Child Welfare League of America (CWLA) 727 15th Street NW, 12th Floor Washington, DC 20005 www.cwla.org	CWLA leads and engages its network of public and private agencies and partners to advance policies, best practices, and collaborative strategies that result in better outcomes for children, youth, and families that are vulnerable.
National Court Appointed Special Advocates (CASA) Association 100 West Harrison Street, North Tower, Suite 500 Seattle, WA 98119 www.casaforchildren.org	The National Court Appointed Special Advocate Association, together with its state and local member programs, supports and promotes court-appointed volunteer advocacy so every abused or neglected child in the United States can be safe, have a permanent home and the opportunity to thrive.
Generations United National Center on Grandfamilies Generations United 1331 H Street NW, Suite 900 Washington, DC 20005 www.gu.org	The mission of Generations United is to improve the lives of children, youth, and older people through intergenerational collaboration, public policies, and programs for the enduring benefit of all.
National Kinship Alliance for Children National Committee of Grandparents for Children's Rights PO Box 85 Ashland, VA 23005 kinshipalliance.org/	The National Committee of Grandparents for Children's Rights is a nationwide network of grandparents, community members, and professionals working together to provide education and support, advocacy, and thought leadership for children, grandparents, and kinship families. This organization's vision is all children having healthy and stable relationships with their grandparents.

ADOPTION/KINSHIP-INFORMED APNS

Despite the goal of adoption/kinship-informed providers, the majority of health care curricula, including nursing's, lack formal education that addresses the needs of these communities and groups (Foli, Forster, & Lim, 2014). This lack of training also applies to those working in the area of adoption and kinship. For example, adoption professionals reported being knowledgeable about depressive symptoms affecting adoptive parents in the postplacement time period; however, 31% were trained in this area (Foli & Gibson, 2011). More specific to nursing, undergraduate nursing students were surveyed on their confidence in rendering care to the adoption triad (Foli et al., 2014). We found that abstract knowledge—what the students thought they knew—was higher than concrete knowledge when presented with clinical vignettes, indicating an overconfidence in students. Conclusions included ways of presenting information about the adoption triad members in the undergraduate curriculum, including panel discussions and reviewing available resources (Foli et al., 2014).

In another study, nurses described wanting to practice in a more informed way and a desire to be adoption-competent in delivering care to the adoption triad (Foli, Schweitzer, & Wells, 2013). A qualitative analysis was performed on brief narratives provided by practicing nurses and their lived experiences with adoption. Four themes emerged from the data: where the personal and professional selves meet (allowing nurses to see the dynamics of adoption from both sides); the paradox of adoption (the loss and joys of adoption); the unique contexts of adoptive families (a recognition of the narratives of those involved with adoption); and reframing nurses' perceptions surrounding adoption (respondents' acknowledgment of the need to improve care for individuals in the adoption triad; Foli et al., 2013). APNs have myriad opportunities to serve these groups, especially as primary care providers, but as with any clinical area, knowledge and clinical context must be offered.

SUMMARY

The loss–healing dichotomy is evident from the history of adoption and the growth in kinship parenting. Molded by history, law, reproductive rights, popular culture, and specific disciplines, unique aspects of adoption and kinship should be understood by APNs. Media presentations of adoption have leaned toward elitism or stigmatization of a "lesser family." These presentations defy the reality that most adoption and kinship families strive to provide a nurturing, safe, and loving home for their children. APNs' awareness of the ideologies that have influenced nontraditional families will enhance patient-centered, holistic care. We have covered the historical, legal, and cultural backgrounds of adoption and kinship; next, we shall move toward specific health care needs.

CHAPTER HIGHLIGHTS

☐ The history of adoption is characterized by shifts in ideology, social mores, principles such as "in the best interest of the child," and the emergence of social work as a profession.

☐ Additional influences of adoption can be found in the aftermath of wars, women's choices regarding motherhood, transracial adoptions, special needs adoptions, globalization, and the shift from domestic orphanages to foster care.

☐ The language surrounding adoption and kinship triads is important because our discourse is shaped by history and social mores, and reflects and creates our current realities.

☐ Today, opposing narratives against hegemonic ideology in adoption practices have been voiced by birth parents and adopted individuals.

☐ Legal guidance in adoption and kinship care has three influences—constitutional law, federal laws, and state statutes with frequent variances among states.

☐ There are three types of adoption: foster care or domestic public adoption, private domestic adoption, and intercountry adoption.

☐ Media depiction of adoption is often skewed, with polarized depictions of elitism (famous parents), highlighting adoptive individuals in news stories unnecessarily, being a second-choice in family building, and sensationalized portrayals of child maltreatment.

☐ Kinship families' legal arrangements vary from legal adoption to informal arrangements decided within families.

☐ Kinship caregiving has a long history in the African American population, and 31% of Black children reside in public or private kinship care.

☐ Legal consent for kinship children's health care may be in the form of affidavits, which do not require birth parents' signatures.

☐ APNs' competence in patient-centered care of adoptive and kinship families can be strengthened through education and clinical experiences.

Questions for Reflection

Following are a few questions to reflect upon. You can use these to start a journal for yourself or in a classroom discussion with peers and the instructor.

1. How does America's history of adoption influence practices and perceptions today? When you read current events in our popular culture, how often is adoption portrayed in a positive light? Have you noted biases before reading this guide?
2. In contrast to adoption, how are kinship families discussed in the popular culture—or are they discussed? Is kinship care overlooked by mainstream society because it is often practiced by underserved, vulnerable groups who are characterized by health disparities?
3. Describe at least one federal or state statute that has influenced adoptive or kinship practices. Now, describe how these practices ultimately impact health care services provided by APNs.
4. How do you view hegemony in adoption and kinship triads? Are they the same or different? Where is the power in discourse, practices, and narratives?

References

Acosta, L. (2013). *Adoption law: United States.* Washington, DC: Library of Congress. Retrieved from www.loc.gov/law/help/adoption-law/unitedstates.php

The Adoption History Project. (2012a). *Indian Adoption Project.* Retrieved from pages.uoregon.edu/adoption/topics/IAP.html

The Adoption History Project. (2012b). *Indian Child Welfare Act.* Retrieved from pages.uoregon.edu/adoption/topics/ICWA.html

Annie E. Casey Foundation. (2012). *Stepping up for kids: What government and communities should do to support kinship families.* Baltimore, MD: Author.

Askren, H. A., & Bloom, K. C. (1999). Postadoptive reactions of the relinquishing mother: A review. *Journal of Obstetric, Gynecologic, and Neonatal Nursing, 28*(4), 395–400.

Baby Scoop Era Research Initiative. (n.d.). *The baby scoop era: Research and inquiry into adoption practice, 1945-1972.* Retrieved from babyscoopera.com

Bastard Nation. (2016). *Bastard Nation mission statement.* Retrieved from bastards.org/mission-statement

Beltran, A. (2013). *Policy brief: State education and health care consent laws.* Washington, DC: Generations United. Retrieved from www.grandfamilies .org/Portals/0/GU%20Policy%20Brief%20February%202014.pdf

Brathwaite, D. O., Bach, B. W., Baxtern, L. A., DeVerniero, R., Hammonds, J. R., Josek, A. M., & Wolf, B. M. (2010). Constructing family: A typology of voluntary kin. *Journal of Social and Personal Relationships, 27,* 388–407.

Brown, S. (2013, September 17). Overseas adoptions rise: For black American children. *CNN.* Retrieved from www.cnn.com/2013/09/16 /world/international-adoption-us-children-adopted-abroad/index.html

Brumble, K., & Kampfe, C. M. (2011). The history of adoption in the United States: A focus on the unique group of intercountry transracial special needs children. *Counseling Psychology Quarterly, 24*(2), 157–162. doi:10.108 0/09515070.2011.586413

Child Welfare Information Gateway. (2016a). *Foster care statistics 2014.* Retrieved from www.childwelfare.gov/pubs/factsheets/foster

Child Welfare Information Gateway. (2016b). *Major Federal legislation concerned with child protection, child welfare, and adoption.* Washington, DC: U.S. Department of Health and Human Services, Children's Bureau.

Child Welfare League of America. (1960). *Child Welfare League of America standards for services to unmarried parents.* New York, NY: Author.

Child Welfare League of America. (2013). Who we are and what we do: Our story. Retrieved from www.cwla.org/about-us/history

Children's Bureau. (2015). History. Retrieved from www.acf.hhs.gov /programs/cb/about/history

Conn, P. (2013). *Adoption: A brief social and cultural history*. New York, NY: Palgrave Macmillan.

The Donaldson Adoption Institute. (2016). Let's adopt reform. Retrieved from www.letsadoptreform.org

Ellis, R. R., & Simmons, T. (2014). Coresident grandparents and their grandchildren: 2012. In *Current population reports* (pp. 20–576). Washington, DC: Census Bureau.

Foli, K. J., Forster, A., & Lim, F. (2014). Student nurses' perceptions of adoption. *Journal of Christian Nursing, 31*(4), 246–251.

Foli, K. J., & Gibson, G. C. (2011). Training "adoption smart" professionals. *Journal of Psychiatric and Mental Health Nursing, 18*(5), 463–467. doi:10.1111/j.1365-2850.2011.01715.x

Foli, K. J., Schweitzer, R., & Wells, C. (2013). The personal and professional: Nurses' lived experiences of adoption. *The American Journal of Maternal /Child Nursing, 38*(2), 79–86. doi:10.1097/NMC.0b013e3182763446

Hegemony. (2016). In *Merriam-Webster online dictionary*. Retrieved from www.merriam-webster.com/dictionary/hegemony

Kahan, M. (2006). "Put up" on platforms: A history of twentieth century adoption policy in the United States. *Journal of Sociology and Social Welfare, 33*(3), 51–72.

Melosh, B. (2002). *Strangers and kin: The American way of adoption*. Cambridge, MA: Harvard University Press.

National Association of Black Social Workers. (1972). *National Association of Black Social Workers position statement on trans-racial adoptions*. Retrieved from c.ymcdn.com/sites/nabsw.org/resource/collection/E1582D77-E4CD-4104 -996A-D42D08F9CA7D/NABSW_Trans-Racial_Adoption_1972_Position_ (b).pdf

National Association of Black Social Workers. (2003). *National Association of Black Social Workers position statement on kinship care position statement*. Retrieved from http://c.ymcdn.com/sites/nabsw.org/resource /collection/E1582D77-E4CD-4104-996A-D42D08F9CA7D/Kinship_ Care_Position_Paper.pdf

National Indian Child Welfare Association. (2015, September). *Setting the record straight: The Indian Child Welfare Act fact sheet*. Retrieved from www.nicwa.org/Indian_Child_Welfare_Act/documents/setting%20 record%20straight.pdf

National Resource Center for Diligent Recruitment. (2016). NRCDR: About us. Retrieved from www.nrcdr.org/about-us

Nelson, M. K. (2014). Whither fictive kin? Or, what's in a name? *Journal of Family Issues, 35*(2), 201–222. doi:10.1177/0192513X12470621

O'Brien, K. M., & Zamostny, K. P. (2003). Understanding adoptive families: An integrative review of empirical research and future direction for counseling psychology. *The Counseling Psychologist, 31*(6), 679–710. doi:10.1177/0011000003258086

Pasztor, E. M. (2015). Kinship care: The history of a name. In K. Phagan-Hansal (Ed.), *The kinship parenting toolbox* (pp. 23–24). Warren, NJ: EMK Press.

Pertman, A. (2000). *Adoption nation: How the adoption revolution is transforming America.* New York, NY: Basic Books.

Rotabi, K. S., & Gibbons, J. L. (2012). Does the Hague Convention on Intercountry Adoption adequately protect orphaned and vulnerable children and their families? *Journal of Child and Family Studies, 21*, 106–119. doi:10.1007/s10826-011-9509-6

Selman, P. (2015). Global statistics for intercountry adoption: Receiving states and states of origin 2003-2013. Retrieved from https://assets.hcch.net/docs/3bead31e-6234-44ae-9f4e-2352b190ca21.pdf

Stack, C. (1983). *All our kin: Strategies for survival in a Black community.* New York, NY: Basic Books.

United Nations, Department of Economic and Social Affairs. (2009). *Child adoptions: Trends and policies.* New York, NY: Author.

U.S. Department of Health and Human Services. (2015, July 9). Trends in foster care and adoption: FY 2005-2014. Retrieved from www.acf.hhs.gov/sites/default/files/cb/trends_fostercare_adoption2014.pdf

U.S. Department of State, Bureau of Consular Affairs. (2015, March 31). *FY 2014 Annual report on intercountry adoption.* Retrieved from travel.state.gov/content/dam/aa/pdfs/fy2014_annual_report.pdf

Vandivere, S., Malm, K., & Radel, L. (2009). *Adoption USA: A chartbook based on the 2007 National Survey of Adoptive Parents.* Washington, DC: U.S. Department of Health and Human Services, Office of the Assistant Secretary for Planning and Evaluation.

II

The Adoption and Kinship Triads

III

The Adoption and Kinship Triads

2

Health Care Needs of Adoptive and Kinship Children

□ □ □ □

PURPOSE OF THE CHAPTER

The purpose of this chapter is to highlight the unique and common health care needs of both adoptive and kinship children and to supplement the comprehensive examination of any pediatric patient. Included are both adoptive and kinship children because there is significant overlap of needs based on the places and spaces they have experienced, including maltreatment and environments of deprivation. Although this is not a full listing of every potential difficulty that these children may present with, the following discussion presents topics that require advanced practice nurses' (APNs') vigilant focus. I divide the chapter into areas of special attention in the immediate evaluation and follow-up of the child, with the caveat that the sum is greater than the parts and that the social unit—the family—should be approached with a holistic perspective.

A second caveat is that for these health care/medical problems, there is no difference between management of adopted and kinship children from that of children in the general population. Similarly, the physical assessment and evaluation is no different in that it should be conducted in a systematic and thorough manner with specific foci. For example, a parasitic infection will have the same treatment protocol for an adopted or nonadopted child. However, for various disorders, the prevalence, risk factors, and presentation may be quite distinct between adopted and kinship children. The APN's focus on certain aspects of the physical examination, treatment plan, coordination of care and referrals to other professionals can and will be unique to these groups of children and adolescents. There are also many references to children who are cared for through the public welfare/foster care system (see also Chapter 9). In the context of this chapter, foster care children represent those individuals who are adopted from the public welfare system or cared for through kinship parenting.

Learning Objectives

At the completion of the chapter, the reader will be able to:

1. Distinguish between adopted/kinship children's overall health risks and those of other children
2. Identify resources from the National Association of Pediatric Nurses and Nurse Practitioners (NAPNAP) and the American Academy of Pediatrics (AAP) to support holistic care rendered by APNs
3. Describe the common acute and long-term care conditions that require health care management in children who are adopted or are in kinship care, including physical, psychosocial, educational, mental health, and developmental conditions
4. Describe follow-up evaluations of children who have been adopted or are in kinship foster care with intentional focus on care coordination, patient-centered care, and medical homes
5. Provide holistic care directly to adoption/kinship children or be able to refer to an appropriate collaborator

OVERALL HEALTH OF ADOPTED CHILDREN

The 2003 National Survey of Children's Health, a nationally representative sample, consisted of 102,353 children, including 2,903 adopted children. The researchers found that adopted children were more likely than biological children to "have special health care needs, current moderate or severe health problems, learning disability, developmental delay or physical impairment, and other mental health difficulties" (p. S54). However, despite these increased needs, adopted children were more likely to be provided with preventive medical care and dental visits, to receive mental health care, and to receive care in a medical home. Additional items were also in the adopted children's favor, and included factors such as consistent health insurance coverage, to be read to daily, or to live in supportive neighborhoods. The authors concluded that the adoptive parents may be doing more than biological parents to provide the needed health care (Bramlett, Radel, & Blumberg, 2007).

The National Survey of Adoptive Parents (NSAP) was an add-on module to the 2007 National Survey of Children's Health that surveyed adoptive parents with 2,737 focal children identified (Vandivere, Malm, & Radel, 2009). Regardless of the type of adoption, this survey revealed that most adopted children are in excellent or very good health (85%). That being stated, 39% of adopted children have special health care needs, in contrast to 19% of all children. They are also more likely to experience moderate or severe health difficulties than children in the general population (26% vs. 10%); and be diagnosed with asthma (19% vs. 13%). The survey also described adopted children performing well on six measures of socio-emotional well-being, such as attachment disorder, depression, attention deficit disorder or attention deficit hyperactivity disorder, or behavior or conduct disorder. The majority of children (88%) ages 6 and older demonstrated positive social behaviors (Vandivere et al., 2009). Over half of the adopted children also demonstrated excellent or very good performance in reading, language arts, and math; however, they were somewhat less likely to be engaged in school than children in general (Vandivere et al., 2009). The reasons for this are unclear.

The National Survey of Adoptive Parents of Children with Special Healthcare Needs (NSAP-SN) survey offered data to support the special needs of adoptive children, which may include children who have been adopted by kinship parents (Bramblett et al., 2010). In the final sample of NSAP-SN (n = 1,003; foster care = 48.5%; private domestic = 33.0%; and international = 18.5%), 76.9% were taking prescription medications; 53.1% had elevated service usage or need; 28.0% had limitation in activity; 27.4% had physical, occupational, or speech therapy; and 50.9% had a behavioral, emotional, or developmental problem; almost half of the children were between 3 and 5 years of age (Bramlett et al., 2010).

Recent attention has been given to families' ongoing challenges during the vulnerable postplacement period, when almost 20% of families engage in family counseling and 57% of adolescents who were adopted from foster care receive mental health services (Smith, 2014; Vandivere et al., 2009). Many adopted children experience adversities early in life; thus, adoptive families often face subsequent challenges that have highlighted a national lack of coordinated postadoption services (Smith, 2010, 2013).

Just as no two children are identical, the paths to adoption—domestic private, domestic public/foster care, and intercountry adoptions—impact the experiences of the adopted persons differently. One type of adoption may typically provide more birth parent and medical information (kinship and foster care), whereas another may provide transfer of parenting at a younger age (domestic private and intercountry). Let us consider them as groups in the discussion that follows.

OBTAINING HEALTH INFORMATION

Children via Private Adoption

Private adoptions in the United States may be arranged with the assistance of an adoption agency or facilitator, or the child may be placed without the use of professionals. When a third party, who is not an adoption agency, brokers the placement of a child, this is called independent adoption. This is the case when members of churches or within families agree that adoptive parent(s) will accept a child from birth parents. Most often, parties know one another. Medical history information, including familial diseases and disorders, usually is available to the adoptive parents.

When an open, private adoption is arranged through an adoption agency, family health history and medical information are obtained. The adoptive family and child are aware of familial risk factors. In contrast, in a confidential adoption, closed records preclude the sharing of this information. Therefore, there is a wide variety of health history available to the APN when domestic private adoptions are arranged.

Children From the Public Welfare System

Placing children from the public welfare system has taken on a new sense of urgency as permanent homes are sought. In 2014, approximately 415,000 children were in foster care across a variety of settings. Of these, 25% or almost 104,000 had the goal of being adopted (Child Welfare Information Gateway, 2016). The website, AdoptUSKids.org, provides a national photo listing of children who are awaiting placement from the foster care system. AdoptUSKids is a project of the U.S. Children's Bureau and is operated through a cooperative agreement with the Adoption Exchange Association. Its mission is to promote adoptions of children in the foster care system and to "support States, Territories, and Tribes to recruit and retain adoptive and foster families" (AdoptUSKids, 2016).

The majority of these children are considered special needs and more difficult to place than children who are not in the foster care system. Exposure to prenatal noxious substances, experiences of maltreatment and trauma, and multisystem health concerns are common. However, stereotypes of children in foster care should be avoided. Behaviors such as fatigue and distractibility may be part of several diagnoses; a skilled APN will be able to understand that diagnosing an adolescent with these symptoms may include depression, auditory processing disorder, attention deficit disorder, chronic fatigue, traumatic stress, iron-deficiency anemia, and others.

Children Adopted From Other Countries

Historically, children who have been received in the United States from other countries often have the least amount of birth information or an optimistic and sometimes inaccurate depiction of their status. In addition to overall medical status, these areas include eating, toileting, and developmental milestones. Another aspect of intercountry adoption is that, in general, there are two types of care offered to children who have been relinquished by birth parents: foster care, where there is usually consistency in caregiving, and orphanage care, which often lacks consistent caregiving and may include sensory and other types of deprivation. Juffer and van IJzendoorn (2005) performed a meta-analysis of international adoption and noted that such adoptees often experience inadequate prenatal and perinatal care, maternal separation, psychological deprivation, insufficient health services, neglect, abuse, and malnutrition in orphanages or poor families before adoption. Findings indicate that international adoptees present with more behavior problems than nonadopted peers and are overrepresented in mental health services. Adoptees with histories of extreme deprivation showed more behavioral problems and externalizing behaviors than adoptees without such adversity. However, the rate of behavior problems is modest, indicating that most international adoptees are well adjusted and experience fewer behavioral problems than domestic adoptees (Juffer & van IJzendoorn, 2005).

In certain countries and with increasing frequency, adoption agencies are encouraging adopted persons to trace their heritage and families within their country of origin. In other instances, with a view to protecting birth mothers' safety, it is not encouraged. An APN will want to understand what type of care the child experienced when assessment is made, as well as the age at adoption and the length of time in institutional care. Overall health status, developmental delays, behaviors related to traumatic events, and neurological behaviors will need to be contextualized to the preplacement care received. Exposure to infectious diseases and toxic agents will also be optimally assessed when this knowledge is applied at assessment.

ASSESSMENT OF THE ADOPTED AND KINSHIP CHILD

The following sections discuss general screenings and assessments of the newly placed child, regardless of the type of adoption (private domestic, public domestic, or intercountry) or whether they are in relative/kinship care. General pediatric screenings will be discussed, and then specific considerations for children who have been placed with adoptive/kinship parents will be presented. This section contains information that will be helpful in follow-up and long-term visits through a medical home for the family and child.

Pediatric Screening: Guidance From the American Academy of Pediatrics

In 2016, the American Academy of Pediatrics (AAP) updated its *Recommendations for Preventive Pediatric Health Care*, or the periodicity schedule. Several updates are included for health care providers assessing pediatric patients (see Exhibit 2.1). The term "pediatrician" is used in

EXHIBIT 2.1

UPDATES TO THE AMERICAN ACADEMY OF PEDIATRICS PERIODICITY SCHEDULE

☐ *The recommendation for routine vision screening at age 18 has been changed to risk-based assessment, based on evidence showing that fewer new vision problems develop in low-risk young adults.*

☐ *To help reduce dental cavities, the top chronic disease affecting young children, a recommendation has been added for fluoride varnish applications from 6 months through 5 years.*

☐ *Pediatricians are advised to use the CRAFFT (Car, Relax, Forget, Friends, Trouble) screening questionnaire as a tool to screen adolescents for drug and alcohol use.*

☐ *Depression screening has been added, with suggested screenings every year from ages 11 through 21, with suicide now a leading cause of death among adolescents.*

☐ *A screening for dyslipidemia, or high blood cholesterol levels, has been added for patients between 9 and 11 years old. The change reflected growing concerns about the growing epidemic of obesity in children.*

☐ *A risk assessment is added at 15 and 30 months for hematocrit or hemoglobin screening to help detect anemia, an iron deficiency.*

☐ *An HIV screen was added for adolescents between 16 and 18 years to address federal statistics showing that one in four new HIV infections occurs in youth ages 13 to 24 years old, and that about 60% of all youth with HIV do not know they are infected.*

☐ *Screen for cervical dysplasia, the presence of precancerous cells on the surface of the cervix, only at 21 years (instead of risk assessment every year from ages 11 through 21).*

☐ *A screening for critical congenital heart disease using pulse oximetry has been added and should be performed in the hospital before newborn discharge.*

Source: AAP (2016a).

Exhibit 2.1 because this summary was issued by the AAP; however, in the context of this chapter, pediatric nurse practitioners (PNPs) and APNs will be also be primary care providers and follow these guidelines. APNs will perform the routine assessments and evaluations on a newly placed child as they would for any other pediatric client.

American Academy of Pediatrics Guidance on Children and Adolescents in Foster Care

In addition to the periodicity table for all pediatric patients, the AAP has an extensive set of resources for the APN in delivering adoption/foster care competent services (see Exhibit 2.2). Although the AAP

EXHIBIT 2.2

THE AMERICAN ACADEMY OF PEDIATRICS RESOURCES ON CHILDREN IN FOSTER CARE

Healthy Foster Care America: Primary Care Tools

Background Documents
☐ *Foster Care Journey*
☐ *Confidentiality Laws Tip Sheet*
☐ *Tips for Working with Children and Teens in Foster Care*
☐ *10 Things Every Pediatrician Should Know About Children in Foster Care*
☐ *Helping Foster and Adoptive Families Cope With Trauma: A Guide for Pediatricians*

Clinical forms
☐ *Health Information Form*
☐ *Health Summary Form*
☐ *Consent to Obtain Confidential Records or Information*
☐ *Consent to Release Confidential Records of Information*
☐ *Referral and Feedback Form*
☐ *Back to Sleep for Babies in Foster Care: Every Time, With Every Caregiver*
☐ *Visit Discharge and Referral Summary for Family*

(continued)

EXHIBIT 2.2 *(continued)*

Other Documents Include

☐ *Office Management*
☐ *Patient Relationship*
☐ *Other Tools and Resources (e.g., Moving to Adulthood: A Handout for Youth Aging out of Foster Care)*

Source: AAP (2016b).

---

designates these as helpful documents for children who reside in or are placed out of foster care, several of these resources are applicable to children who have been placed from other countries. Each document is a source of information unique to this population of children and is easily consumed and helpful in contextualizing the care of children who have been removed from their birth parents' homes. Clinical forms should be adapted to the organization in which the APN practices. One resource is of particular note: At almost 200 pages, *Fostering Health: Health Care for Children and Adolescents in Foster Care* (AAP, 2005) describes provisions of care because "[c]hildren and adolescents in foster care have a higher prevalence of physical, developmental, dental, and behavioral health conditions than any other group of children" (p. ix). PNPs are specifically included as primary care providers referenced in this manual.

EVALUATION OF THE ADOPTED AND KINSHIP CHILD

Within the medical profession is a subspecialty called "adoption medicine." The book *Adoption Medicine: Caring for Children and Families* was published in 2014 by the AAP and consolidated the knowledge needed to provide medical care to pediatric patients who had been adopted (Mason, Johnson, & Prock, 2014). In further recognition of this specialty area and through their Council on Foster Care, Adoption, and Kinship Care, the AAP has created a state-by-state list of pediatricians who focus on adoption, foster care, and kinship care (see aap.org). Many larger cities, especially those with universities, will also have international adoption clinics with physicians and other health care providers who are specialists in the evaluation and care of children who have been adopted from other countries and, increasingly, from domestic and foster care adoptions. APNs may find these resources useful when seeking referrals for patients who have been evaluated and require follow-up services.

INITIAL EVALUATION

Timing of Initial Evaluation

For recently placed internationally adopted children, unless there is an acute illness, the AAP recommends that the initial evaluation occur within 3 weeks of the child's arrival home (Schulte & Springer, 2014). A follow-up should be performed 4 to 6 weeks after this initial evaluation (Schulte & Springer, 2014). For children who are removed from their homes and placed in kinship (relative placement through the child welfare system) or foster care, evaluations are mandated by state laws, which vary among states. Limits are placed on the timing of the initial evaluation, with some states requiring the child to be assessed within 24 hours to as long as 10 days postremoval from the home. The AAP recommends evaluation within 72 hours of placement, within 24 hours if abuse is suspected (Council on Foster Care, Adoption and Kinship Care, Committee on Adolescence, & Council on Early Childhood, 2015). Clearly, the closer the evaluation is to the time of removal from the home, the more accurate the assessment will be in determining past maltreatment. Documentation of suspected physical and sexual abuse should be a priority in the assessment.

Content of Initial Evaluation

Health History

A comprehensive gathering of medical history and physical examination findings of the child or adolescent needs to be conducted at the initial evaluation. Obtaining an accurate and current medical and health history for children who are removed from their homes—for any reason—can prove to be challenging. At times, children who are adopted from other countries will have accompanying health information, documents, or videotapes. A specialist in adoption medicine should review these records to advise on accuracy and findings. In my own personal experience, we received a 45-second video of a small baby in a very loud orphanage who had fearful eyes and slowly brought her thumb to her mouth in a self-soothing way. In 45 seconds, we caught a brief view into her world and what she needed. The paperwork grossly overestimated this child's (my daughter's) dietary intake and physical development. Only when we treated her iron deficiency were we able to see her true personality present itself. For other children, videos may be substantially longer, and when shown to an adoption medicine specialist, can offer families some information into the potential needs of the child being adopted.

When a child is removed from the home because of maltreatment, the case worker attempts to complete a medical history, but this is not always possible because of tension at the time of removal. If the birth parent is also incapacitated by illness, substance use, or other cognitive deficits, a health history will be difficult to record because the birth parent may be unable to comprehend the questions. The immediate safety and well-being of the child is a priority for the case worker who is charged with removing the child from the environment. The interactions between the birth parents and the case workers may be acrimonious, and will preclude case workers from being able to collect and, therefore, communicate health information. At times, incomplete information is passed through the child welfare system and uncovered later in the process. For example, foster parents who adopted a medically fragile child were told that a minor and repairable physical abnormality was the extent of the medical needs. As they underwent training to care for the child, they discovered a network of over a dozen health care providers and several unknown complex needs. This is not uncommon, and medical, mental health, and developmental needs may arise after the child is in care or a consistent caregiver begins to parent the child.

Safe-Haven babies, which we discuss in Chapter 3, have been brought to and left in designated and approved areas soon after birth. Typically, there is no prenatal, birth, health, or medical information accompanying these babies, and, therefore, no information is available to their new caretakers. Kinship parents also may be unaware of what transpired during the time the child was under the care of the birth parents. One relative discovered that the child, who had normal cognitive functioning, had not been toilet trained until he was 8 years old. At other times, the kinship parent "may not want to know" the health history because it is too painful to learn the negative experiences the child has endured.

Court-appointed special advocates (CASA) volunteers, school counselors, foster parents, and others may be able to provide some history given that they communicate with birth parents and the child. Requests for available records should be made to obtain a comprehensive health history. Understanding the child's/adolescent's history may be a process that evolves over time rather than a task that is considered complete after the initial evaluation. The interview process with the child/adolescent also offers the potential for rich information to help understand past experiences and needs, as well as priorities of the individual within the family dynamic. Even young children may be able to report health-related signs and symptoms, and traumatic events in their lives.

Prenatal exposure to toxic substances and illicit drugs by the birth mother may also be unknown or difficult to ascertain. However, current and past medications prescribed for the child/adolescent play an important role in taking a current health status inventory. As noted earlier, almost 80% of adopted children with special needs were being prescribed medications (Bramblett et al., 2010). Various placements with different systems of care may result in an incomplete inventory of current medications. Adverse and side effects to these medications also need to be carefully assessed by the APN. Further, an inventory of bathing and toileting patterns should be assessed as these may relate to areas of sleep/rest, nutrition, infectious diseases, and past traumas.

The APN should also be aware that adoptive and kinship parents may cope with the unexpected needs of their children in different ways. We discuss parental postadoption depression in Chapter 4, but it should be noted that parents may be faced with significant psychological, emotional, social, and financial challenges as a result of unknown medical and behavioral needs of their newly adopted/placed children. APNs should assess how parents are adapting to new information and disclosures that were unanticipated before placement. Supporting parents in meeting these needs will also mean the APN views the family as a system, with partners and siblings in the home. Family members' needs should be assessed and support offered through therapeutic communication, education, and, when needed, referrals.

Physical Examination

In addition to the physical assessment conducted for *any* child or adolescent, there are specific areas that are pertinent to children who have been adopted or placed in kinship care (Jones & Committee on Early Childhood, Adoption and Dependent Care, 2012). Key assessments as part of the physical examination for adopted children are listed in Table 2.1. For older children and adolescents, screening for depression and suicidal ideation is also warranted. We discuss each of these areas in more depth in the following.

TABLE 2.1 *Components of the Comprehensive Physical Examination for Adopted and Kinship Children*

☐ Vital signs (temperature, pulse, respiratory rate, blood pressure [starting at age 3 years])

☐ Growth points, including length or height, weight, head circumference (on all children up to age 2 years). Data should be plotted on World Health Organization's growth charts, along with comparison with any measurements previously obtained. Body mass index (BMI) should be calculated and plotted on all children age 2 years and older

    ○ Note signs of poor nutrition or malnutrition (secondary to nutritional intake, enteric infections [intestinal parasites], HIV infection, or obesity [empty calories, lack of protein])

☐ Complete physical examination, with emphasis on the following areas:

  ■ Respiratory tract

    ○ Upper respiratory tract infections (including pertussis, severe acute respiratory tract infections [SARS])

    ○ Tuberculosis (usually asymptomatic; however, infants may present with mild cough and dyspnea)

  ■ Skin examination

    ○ Identify infectious diseases, rashes (including rash associated with measles), or infestations, including scabies, lice, cutaneous fungus, and impetigo

    ○ Identify and document any congenital skin abnormalities, including hemangiomas, nevi, and blue macules of infancy (usually seen in children of Asian, African, or Hispanic ethnicity)

    ○ Identify and document bruises or scars that may have resulted from previous abuse or previous immunization

    ○ Pale mucous membranes, lips, or nail bed to assess for anemia

  ■ Congenital disorders examination

    ○ Identify cardiac abnormalities

    ○ Note evidence of cleft lip and/or palate

  ■ Careful genitalia examination (including the anus) should be performed to identify any abnormality suspicious for prior sexual abuse or genital cutting

    ○ Testing for sexually transmitted diseases should be performed with any suspicion of abuse or if the child/adolescent is sexually active

---

(continued)

TABLE 2.1   *Components of the Comprehensive Physical Examination for Adopted and Kinship Children (continued)*

- Musculoskeletal examination, with an emphasis on bone deformities caused by vitamin deficiencies (e.g., rickets-bowing of the distal tibiae), and other conditions such as hypotonia
- Neurological examination, with emphasis on developmental and neurological abnormalities
  - Signs of central and autonomic nervous system withdrawal from prenatal substances, such as opioids in infants
  - Screen for depression/suicidal ideation in older children and adolescents
- Documentation should include child's/adolescent's tolerance to the examination, including exaggerated or muted reactions to the physical examination (which may be related to potential trauma reminders [disrobing, being touched, etc.]), sensory issues, or other behavioral/developmental problems. Translators should be available to assist the child in understanding the physical assessment.

Adapted from Jones and Committee on Early Childhood, Adoption and Dependent Care (2012); Kim and Staat (2004).

SPECIFIC PHYSICAL NEEDS

Sleep and Rest

One of the most commonly overlooked areas to assess is sleep hygiene and the sleep–wake cycles of children who have been adopted or under kinship care. Parents often remark that their child, despite seeming independent and content during the day, suffers from night terrors and nightmares (and therefore, the adults' sleep is often of poor quality). Often, children refuse to sleep alone and will insist on using a family bed/shared bed/cosleeping, a controversial topic in health care. The AAP recommends room sharing; however, it does not recommend cosleeping arrangements in view of the risks of entrapment and suffocation. Some parents allow a child to sleep on a pallet next to their bed at night in order to feel safe.

Children's sleep–wake cycle will need to be assessed carefully because symptoms of fatigue may be applicable to several diagnoses. In children who are overweight or obese, which may be assessed in children who have sedentary lives and consume high-calorie, poor nutrient, processed foods, sleep apnea should be evaluated through a sleep study. Assumptions that a quiet environment is needed for the child to sleep may not be accurate. Our daughter, who spent the first months of her life in an orphanage, could not sleep without background noise, which is what she was accustomed to in the nursery. Children who are newly adopted may also experience sleep disturbances as they acclimate to their new surroundings and recover from time zone differences (after intercountry travel). Past trauma can also account for night terrors and disruptions in sleep. One kinship mother ensured that the nightlight was on for her granddaughter, who had suffered abuse and often awakened during the night seeking her comfort.

The literature also points to sleep problems being present in adopted children: 52% of parents reported that their children ($n = 240$) who were adopted from China experienced sleep problems; however, only 9% were considered significant (Rettig & McCarthy-Rettig, 2006). In a sample of children diagnosed with autistism spectrum disorders, adopted children experienced significantly higher sleep disturbances than nonadopted children (Ezell, Shui, Sanders, & Veenstra-VanderWeele, 2016). In addition to a history, physical signs are important to note, which may lead an APN to further explore sleep disruptions and problems. Asymmetrical tympanic membrane temperatures (higher left than right) have been associated with increased sleep problems in toddlers who were adopted from China (Damsteegt, van IJzendoom, Out, & Bakermans-Kranenburg, 2014).

Nutrition and Growth

Malnutrition should be assessed closely for its relationship to fine and gross motor development, as well as cognitive and psychosocial development. Specific nutrient and vitamin deficiencies may be present (e.g., calcium, vitamin D, phosphorus). Although the evidence often points to the lack of nutrition in children who have been placed from developing countries, I have spoken to many foster and kinship parents who disclosed that their children lacked proper and adequate nutrition. Indeed, anecdotal reports of children in the United States who have been locked in rooms and allowed one meal per day have been conveyed. When I present the trauma-informed parenting classes for kinship parents, I also bring healthy, copious amounts of food for the children, who will often overeat (if not appropriately supervised) and hoard food for later. Survival skills, such as taking food when it is available, have created these behaviors. Parents report hoarding is a common behavior, and hiding the food in socks, shoes, "anywhere they can think of," is typical of children who have experienced hunger on a continual basis. Educating parents on hoarding is needed: Advising parents to allow children to take a snack for later will offer the child a sense of control and safety, both desperately needed by children who have experienced trauma. Paradoxically, obesity in children from the public welfare system is not uncommon and is due to lack of exercise and poor-quality diets (Schulte & Springer, 2014).

For children who have been adopted internationally, the length of time spent in the institution and age at adoption are important to note. APNs should use the appropriate growth charts for children who have been adopted from other countries. The World Health Organization, Multicentre Growth Reference Study Group (2006) updated standard measurements for children under 5 years of age: weight-for-length/height; weight-for-age; length/height-for-age; and body mass index (BMI)-for-age. For children over 5 years, the Centers for Disease Control and Prevention (CDC) growth charts can be used as a point of comparison (Kuczmarski et al., 2000).

For all children, anthropometric measurement should be carefully assessed, including upright or recumbent height measurements, depending on the age of the child; weight; and head circumference. Laboratory values should also be assessed, including a complete blood count, with a close examination of iron, calcium, iodine, and vitamin D values. Stool samples should also be collected to rule out parasites. Examinations of iron levels of intercountry adopted children reveal the potential effects of micronutrient deficiency on development (Doom et al., 2014; Fuglestad et al., 2013). Iron deficiency (ID) and length of deprivation experienced by 55 children ages 17 to 36 months and adopted from institutions around the world (e.g., Africa, Asia, Eastern Europe, and Latin America) were studied (Doom et al., 2014). Findings included 11 children with low hemoglobin levels and 16 additional children with ID and one or two abnormal indices; 28 children had normal iron levels. Lower IQ scores and executive function performance were related to ID at adoption and longer lengths of care in institutions (Doom et al., 2014). Fuglestad et al. (2013) found hyperactivity in children with ID and recommended screening for ID during the first 6 months postadoption.

APNs should also be aware that certain ethnicities have slightly lower hemoglobin levels because of genetic traits. For example, individuals from Asia, the Middle East, Africa, and Eastern Europe are more prone to thalassemia and face a higher risk of carrying the sickle cell gene. Differentiating between nutrition-based ID and other conditions that cause anemia is important when assessing children who are adopted or in kinship care.

Oral/Dental Health

In all children, dental caries is the most common chronic condition (AAP [Section on Oral Health], 2014). The lack of oral health has been cited repeatedly as a common need in adopted and kinship children. The lack of preventive oral health and the deficit of parental instruction surrounding dental hygiene contribute to this problem. An additional risk factor is the transmission of *Streptococcus mutans* from the mother with dental decay to the child (AAP [Section on Oral Health], 2014). Referral to a dentist is often warranted with education to the child/ adolescent and parent on preventive health and the risks of untreated dental caries. Education should stress the importance of hygiene and potential complications stemming from the lack of care. The Fostering Connections to Success and Increasing Adoptions Act of 2008 also specifies that children in foster care have a coordinated plan for dental health. For all children, the application of toothpaste (a smear until age 3 and then pea size) and dental fluoride varnish every 3 to 6 months (from the first tooth emergence) is now recommended by the AAP until the child receives treatment in a dental home (Clark, Slayton, & Section on Oral Health, 2014). Fluoride varnish may be administered by both dental and nondental providers (as approved by state law), and, thus, may be applied by APNs in primary care settings.

Cleft lip and/or palate is also not uncommon in children who are adopted. These facial abnormalities are a result of incomplete closure of facial structures prior to birth. The APN will note the areas that are affected (lip, palate, unilateral, bilateral, and so forth). The provider will also note how long the cleft lip or palate has been unrepaired and if it is likely to have affected nutritional intake. Referral to appropriate specialists, including cleft and craniofacial surgeons, speech/language therapists, and orthodontists is required. Education on feeding techniques will need to be offered to the parents to ensure proper nutritional intake.

Infectious Diseases and Exposure to Lead

Infectious diseases such as human immunodeficiency virus (HIV); tuberculosis; hepatitis A, B, and C; syphilis; herpes simplex; cytomegalovirus; toxoplasmosis; and parasitic infestations (intestinal and skin) often occur more frequently in these groups of children—and children should be screened via laboratory tests accordingly. In addition, sexually transmitted diseases will need to be assessed, particularly if the child has a history of sexual abuse or is sexually active. If immunization records are incomplete, titers may need to be drawn to determine coverage. "Catch up" immunization schedules may need to be employed if the child has not received timely care. Tuberculosis screening through a purified protein derivative (PPD) test should be administered to children 3 months and older (AAP, 2005).

Lead exposure is not uncommon in these groups, and levels should be drawn for children 6 months to 6 years and for older children based on environmental history (AAP, 2005). APNs should consult *The Red Book* (AAP [Committee on Infectious Diseases], 2015), which highlights infectious disease considerations for children who are adopted internationally and for refugee and immigrant children.

NOXIOUS SUBSTANCE EXPOSURE

The National Center on Substance Abuse and Child Welfare (n.d.) reported that between 67% and 75% of the cases in which a child had been removed from the home involved parental substance abuse. The estimated total number of children who are affected by parental substance use is significant. Estimates are that more than seven million children, born in the United States and younger than 18 years, may have endured parental substance use that resulted in the loss of custody (Coles, 2014). Children who have been exposed to tobacco, alcohol, marijuana, opioids, cocaine, methamphetamine, and other substances may present with abnormal physical, cognitive, and developmental statuses. Exposure may be prenatal, postnatal, or as a child/adolescent living in a home where the manufacturing of drugs is ongoing. Polysubstance abuse is not uncommon in birth mothers and, whenever possible, should be noted in the health history.

Methamphetamine Exposure

Risks for children in homes with parents who use methamphetamine include not only exposure, but ingestion. Children taken from such a home will be part of a legal chain of evidence, and urine and hair samples should be taken if not previously obtained (McGuinness & Pollack, 2008). Although the research is growing, studies to date indicate that a variety of outcomes are possible for children prenatally exposed to methamphetamine and include deficiencies in brain structure, lower birth weight and gestational size, and potential neurobehavioral differences (Hayward, DePanfilis, & Woodruff, 2010; McGuinness & Pollack, 2008). Older children may have physical (e.g., asthma), cognitive (e.g., learning disabilities), and emotional/social difficulties (e.g., antisocial behaviors) because of either exposure or the environment of parental substance abuse (Hayward et al., 2010).

Neonatal Abstinence Syndrome

Infants who have been prenatally exposed to opioids are often diagnosed with neonatal abstinence syndrome (NAS) while still in the hospital, but this may not always be the case. Symptoms can arise up to 4 weeks after birth (Krandall & Gartner, 1974). Several systems in the body are affected and include the central nervous system (CNS), autonomic nervous system, gastrointestinal tract, and respiratory system (Jones & Fielder, 2015). Left untreated, there is significant risk of morbidity and mortality. Treatment consists of hospitalization, pharmacological intervention, and intense monitoring. Therefore, APNs in both acute and primary care settings may encounter infants who are withdrawing from prenatal exposure.

Jones and Fielder (2015) reviewed NAS from current and historical perspectives. They found that assessment and management of NAS accelerated as a result of the Neonatal Abstinence Scoring System (NASS) developed by Finnegan and colleagues in 1975 (Finnegan, Connaughton, Kron, & Emich, 1975). The tool contains 20 of the most common signs of neonatal withdrawal and is the most widely used tool today. However, there are weaknesses: training required to administer, judgment required among raters, differential weighting of items, and lack of studies that have reported the sensitivity and specificity of the tool (Jones & Fielder, 2015). There are modifications of the NASS (e.g., Jansson, Velez, & Harrow, 2009), as well as other tools that have been developed to determine the extent of symptoms related to NAS. Continued research is needed in assessing these tools as well as shorter, more efficient assessments of NAS (Jones & Fielder, 2015).

Fetal Alcohol Spectrum Disorders

Alcohol intake by pregnant women can result in fetal alcohol spectrum disorders (FASDs). The three major types of FASDs are fetal alcohol syndrome (FAS); alcohol-related neurodevelopmental disorder (ARND); and alcohol-related birth defects (ARBD). Children with FAS, the most severe outcome of prenatal alcohol exposure, present with facial dysphorphia: a smooth philtrum (the ridge between the upper lip and nose), thin vermillion border, and small palpebral fissures. Children with FAS also have growth retardation, and CNS disorders. All three facial abnormalities, documented stunted growth, and documented CNS abnormalities are required for a diagnosis of FAS (Bertrand et al., 2004). In ARND, children may exhibit intellectual difficulties and problems with learning, impulse control, memory, attention, and judgment. Lastly, children with ARBD may have problems with their heart, kidneys, bones, or with their hearing (CDC, 2015).

Binge drinking by pregnant women affects child cognition, and there is no known safe amount of alcohol for pregnant women to consume (Flak et al., 2014). Yet alcohol intake by pregnant women continues, and FASDs often go undetected. Chasnoff, Wells, and King (2015) examined 547 foster and adopted children who had undergone a multidisciplinary diagnostic evaluation. Of those children who were evaluated, 156 met the criteria for FASD, 125 had never been diagnosed, and 10 children who had been diagnosed along the spectrum had their diagnoses changed. In total, 86.5% of the children with FASD had never been diagnosed or had been misdiagnosed (Chasnoff et al., 2015).

Figure 2.1 outlines the framework for FAS diagnosis and services that APNs can use when evaluating children who present with medical history or physical presentation triggers that require additional assessment. A patient-centered plan of services with a collaborating team of professionals is highlighted (Bertrand et al., 2004).

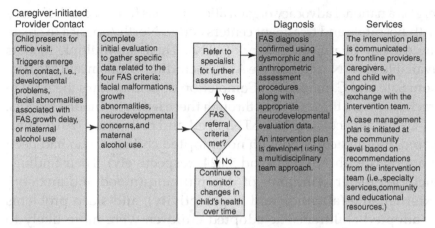

FIGURE 2.1   *Framework for fetal alcohol syndrom diagnosis and services.*
Source: Bertrand et al. (2004).

Developmental/Neurodevelopmental/Behavioral Needs

Developmental delays and neurodevelopmental abnormalities may be attributed to a variety of etiologies (e.g., prenatal exposure to toxic substances, sensory deprivation, malnutrition, and genetic factors). A commonly used tool by pediatric primary care providers is the Denver II Developmental Screening Test (Denver II; Frankenburg, Dodds, Archer, Shapiro, & Bresnick, 1992). The Denver II screens infants and young children (1 month to 6 years) for possible developmental issues, with the provider performing surveillance screenings at every visit. The APN will refer to specialists to determine the extent of the delay and behavioral need. Mental health issues and the adopted individual are discussed in more depth in Chapter 5.

Autism Spectrum Disorder

As most APNs are aware, the separate diagnoses of autism disorder, pervasive developmental disorder not otherwise specified (PDD-NOS), and Asperger's syndrome are now diagnosed under autism spectrum disorder (ASD; CDC, 2016). The prevalence of ASD rose by 123% between 2002 and 2010; however, prevalence rates have been stable between 2010 and 2012 (CDC, 2016). These statistics were collected through the CDC's Autism and Developmental Disabilities Monitoring (ADDM) network on 8-year-old children, who have by this age been identified as needing services. Autism Speaks® (2016; autismspeaks

.org) is a national advocacy organization that has formed collaborations with hospitals and treatment centers across North America to create the Autism Treatment Network (ATN). There are multiple toolkits available to APNs through the ATN, including "Autism and Medication: Safe and Careful Use." Completion of fields allows the ATN to track users and those reached through these federally funded toolkits.

Using data collected by ATN, Ezell and colleagues (2016) compared adopted children with nonadopted children who had been diagnosed with ASD (163 and 5,624, respectively). Their findings include greater symptoms of internalizing (mood and anxiety), externalizing (attention and hyperactivity), and sleep problems in adopted children. The adopted children were more likely to receive psychotropic medications and be diagnosed with PDD-NOS, considered a diagnostic subtype, despite no difference on symptom measures (*Diagnostic and Statistical Manual of Mental Disorders, fourth edition* [*DSM-IV*] criteria were used). Of note, a higher proportion of the adopted children were female, in contrast to the overall population profile of ASD children, and the adopted children were diagnosed at a later age than their nonadopted counterparts (Ezell et al., 2016).

APNs should be aware of these differences and the higher prevalence of behavioral issues in adopted children with ASD, which may delay diagnosis. Female adopted children should also be closely screened for ASD symptoms. An AAP-endorsed screening tool is the Modified Checklist for Autism in Toddlers, Revised with Follow Up (M-CHAT-R/F™; Robins, Fein, & Barton, 2009; Robins et al., 2014). In addition to developmental surveillance at each visit, APNs utilize this tool for developmental screenings for all children at the recommended points, 18 and 24 months, to screen for ASDs (Johnson & Myers, 2007). Referral for an accurate diagnosis to a behavioral pediatrician should be done in the provider's area. Future research is needed to provide elucidation as to whether factors such as birth parent history, age at adoption, and early childhood experiences are related to ASD symptoms in adopted children (Ezell et al., 2016).

Attention Deficit Hyperactivity Disorder

Attention deficit hyperactivity disorder (ADHD) is considered to be familial in nature affecting a higher proportion of adopted children than the general population (Simmel, Brooks, Barth, & Hinshaw, 2001). Parental reports of approximately 800 adopted youth found that the 21.8% had ADHD symptomatology (Simmel et al., 2001), compared with 5% of children across cultures (American Psychiatric Association [APA], 2013). This evidence is tempered with findings that support adoptive family cohesion and adaptability as mediators to adopted youth's ADHD symptoms (Crea, Chan, & Barth, 2013). APNs will need to use a holistic approach when using prescriptive authority and balance this with behavioral modifications to manage the child/adolescent ADHD symptoms.

Communication Disorders

Children who have been adopted from other countries or who experienced maltreatment (abuse and/or neglect) by birth parents in the United States may have to overcome several communication challenges due to exposure to language barriers, toxins, poor health care, trauma, and deprivation. These communication disorders may be familial in nature, part of a learning disability, a comorbid disorder (e.g., ASD), or part of a physical problem. For example, otitis media infections that have gone untreated may result in hearing loss, poor balance, language impairment, and desensitization to pain. APNs should use standardized measures to assess language development based on the child's age.

Exposure to institutional care (routinized care, multiple caregivers, grouped with other children), adoption at an older age, and length of exposure to institutional care have been considered key elements affecting child outcomes in internationally adopted children. There is extensive literature in speech-language-and-hearing sciences, medicine, and nursing that describes these variables and their relationships to negative outcomes. One study by Rakhlin et al. (2015) described the effects of such institutionalized care by comparing internationally adopted children from Russia ($n = 74$) with birth children ($n = 55$) and matched them by age and gender (mean age was 5 years); the children were assessed at two time points (initial assessment and 1 year later; Rakhlin et al., 2015). Two of the notable findings were that, even when other variables were controlled for, the length of time in institutionalized care held the most robust association with child outcomes, and the majority of the internationally adopted children were able to reach normative standards between 1 and 2 years postadoption (Rakhlin et al., 2015).

APNs in primary care often are one of the first points of contact with adoptive and kinship parents who may be concerned about language development. Attention to both receptive and expressive communication is important to assess and document (see also Learning Disabilities section later in this chapter for communication disorders). APNs assess the developmental speech milestones that a child should achieve by age. For example, by 2 years of age, a child should be able to put 2- to 3-word sentences together, name objects, and have speech that is understood by most family members. When the APN notes concern, referrals to agencies that specialize in early intervention should be done to screen children 3 years of age and under for speech and developmental issues. For children who are school age, a referral should be made to the local school district for a speech evaluation. All children with speech concerns should be referred to audiology for a hearing evaluation (see also the section on central auditory processing disorders [CAPD] later in this chapter).

Learning Disabilities/Differences

Many individuals and parents who are enmeshed in the learning disabilities communities prefer the term "learning differences" over "learning disabilities." The rationale for this language is to emphasize that learning can take place for children who process information differently. For the purposes of this discussion, however, we will use the term "learning disabilities." Learning disabilities take many forms, from difficulty in reading to listening to communicating. One of the variables associated with increased odds of having learning disabilities is being adopted (Altarac & Saroha, 2007). Although APNs may believe that learning disabilities lie outside their knowledge base and expertise, the truth is that families approach their primary health care providers when seeking help in dealing with issues that cross over into the educational realm, such as learning disabilities. It is important for APNs to be comfortable and familiar with the interface between the medical/health care and educational realms.

In view of the key role that primary health providers play, one major resource for medical professionals is the "LD Navigator." Through support from the Robert Wood Johnson Foundation, the National Center for Learning Disabilities collaborated with the AAP and the National Association of Pediatric Nurses and Nurse Practitioners (NAPNAP) and created an online toolkit for pediatric health care providers (National Center for Learning Disabilities, 2016). The LD Navigator is specifically designed for pediatric health care providers to disseminate useful information to both parents and patients:

> The LD Navigator is like a compass to guide pediatric health-care professionals as they navigate the complex seas of learning disabilities. It includes up-to-date information about screening, evaluation, classification and treatment, as well as addressing sensitive and important concerns over time of both the parents and the youth with a learning disability. (LD Navigator, 2013a)

This resource, the LD Navigator, presents information that is of critical use to pediatric patients who are experiencing learning disabilities. The bridge between medical/health care services and educational support services has to be successfully crossed in order for parents to effectively receive services for their children. For example, medical terminology describes deficits, whereas educational language emphasizes strengths and weaknesses (LD Navigator, 2013b). In order for parents to successfully approach and obtain services, the APN needs to understand the importance of the lexicon and how to bridge the language used in the *Diagnostic and Statistical Manual of Mental Disorders* (fifth edition; APA, 2013) with the federal law governing services called the Individuals with Disabilities Education Act (IDEA). The LD Navigator is an excellent resource that delivers the foundation and tools needed for APNs to dialogue with children and parents from adoptive and kinship families who may be struggling.

Learning disabilities are neurological disorders that impact the reception, processing, and communication of information. Common learning differences include dyslexia (reading disability), dysgraphia (writing disability), and dyscalculia (learning disability in mathematics). There are also coexisting disabilities that affect a child's and adolescent's educational performance. Schools need to address all of the disabilities that the child/adolescent is diagnosed with, including dyspraxia (disorder that0 affects motor skill development), difficulties with executive functioning (related to planning, organizing, management of time and space), which is often diagnosed by a neuropsychologist, and ADHD, a neurobiological disorder that was discussed earlier in relation to adoption.

Additional coexisting disabilities include auditory processing disorders (also called central auditory processing disorders, or CAPD). CAPD is defined, in a broad sense, by how efficiently and effectively the CNS processes sounds (LD Navigator, 2013b). Children may have comorbid communication disorders; however, peripheral hearing may test as normal. Federal law does not include CAPD as a learning disability, and the diagnosis of CAPD is performed by an audiologist who is specifically trained in the testing of CAPD (a routine hearing test will not determine whether the child has CAPD). The symptoms of CAPD can mimic several learning disabilities (e.g., reading and comprehension difficulties), as well as ADHD (e.g., distraction, inattention, saying, "uh?" frequently, not following directions) (American Speech-Language-Hearing Association, 2005). The APN should be aware of CAPD, particularly when children and adolescents may not be responding to interventions designed to manage other disorders.

Visual processing disorder is also not considered a learning disability under federal law; however, it impacts the individual's ability to distinguish among letters, shapes, colors, patterns, and objects (LD Navigator, 2013b). Again, APNs should understand that a routine eye test may be unable to detect this disorder, but learning and performance may be impacted.

Our society seems to raise the bar higher and higher for career success, and favors individuals with verbal skills. Children and adolescents who struggle with learning differences may be subject to myths and stereotypes. APNs need to advocate for children with suspected learning and communication difficulties to be evaluated through the school district and to have an Individualized Education Plans (IEPs) appropriately put in place if needed. Families need to be informed of the facts surrounding LDs (see Table 2.2). Acceptance, hope, education, and appropriate referrals can make a difference in a child's success or failure. Adoptive and kinship parents and children

TABLE 2.2 *Dispelling Myths Surrounding Individuals With Learning Disabilities (LDs)*

Myth	Fact
People with LD are not intelligent.	People with LD have average or above-average intelligence.
People with LD are lazy and unmotivated.	People with LD work harder and longer than most people to get through the day.
Dyslexia and LD are the same disorder.	Dyslexia is only one type of LD. It is language-based and affects reading, writing, and other communication skills. LD is the umbrella term.
LD only affects children. Adults outgrow LD.	LD lasts throughout an individual's lifetime, but individuals with LD can lead adaptive strategies and skills, and access reasonable accommodations.
LD only affects school achievement and skills.	LD can also affect social, career, and life-management skills.
Learning disabilities are all the same.	Learning disabilities vary greatly from person to person, and combine with other difficulties differently, as well.
Boys are affected by LD more than girls.	There is no gender difference in the incidence of LD. However, boys are diagnosed two times as often, perhaps because of differences in behavior between girls and boys.
Giving LD students accommodations and modifications in school gives them an unfair advantage over other students.	Students with LD must meet the same academic standards as their peers. Their accommodations merely 'level the playing field' so they can participate and achieve equally.

Source: Learning Disabilities Navigator. (2013a). Reprinted with permission. For more information, visit ldnavigator.ncld.org.

can be empowered to advocate for themselves once their health care and learning needs are fully evaluated.

SENSORY ISSUES

Hearing and Vision

Screening for normal hearing and vision is often absent from a child's history. Children ages 3 years and older should have vision and hearing screenings (AAP, 2005). The APN should refer or screen children under 3 years of age on the basis of history or physical examination presentation.

Sensory Processing Disorder

Upon evaluation, a parent might confide to an APN: "He can't stand to be touched. He won't let me hold him;" "He has to have something in his hand all the time;" "She'll gag on scrambled eggs;" or "He gets overloaded very quickly in a crowded room." All of these types of symptoms may be related to an inability to process sensory information, an aspect of self-regulation. Some children exhibit signs of both sensory aversion and sensory seeking behaviors. APNs are in an influential position when interacting with parents who have recently adopted or become caregivers for children who may have difficulties with sensory stimulation. For example, a parent who reports that the child cannot stand to be hugged may mistakenly interpret this to be a rejection of affection. One parent reported that with her previous children, she and they had enjoyed massages, which had helped the infants/children to relax and fall asleep. With the adopted child, however, it only increased the child's agitation, leaving the mother frustrated and confused: What the mother had considered a successful parenting practice was now increasing her daughter's discomfort and the mother's feelings of being rejected. APNs can explain that sensory processing has many facets that, when understood, can support parent–child interactions.

Although not included in the *Diagnostic and Statistical Manual of Mental Disorders* (fifth edition; APA, 2013), the idea of sensory integrative dysfunction (SID) was introduced by Jean Ayres in the 1960s (1963, 1965). Within the purview of occupational therapists, SID or sensory processing disorder (SPD) has been in the literature of early child development since Ayres' seminal work. Additionally, *The Out-of-Sync Child* (Kranowitz, 2005) reached into the lay population with descriptions of the needs of children who either sought out or were repelled by sensory information. SID/SPD has been found to be a comorbid condition with other disorders, such as ASD.

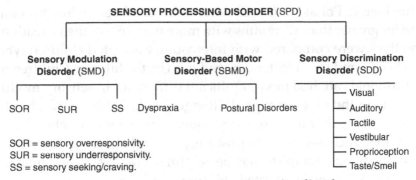

FIGURE 2.2   *A proposed nosology for sensory processing disorder.*
Source: Miller, Anzalone, Lane, Cermak, and Osten (2007). Reprinted with permission from the American Occupational Therapy Association.

Different subtypes of SID/SPD have been discussed:

- Pattern 1: Sensory Modulation Disorder, in which the individual has difficulty responding to the stimuli in a graded manner (hypersensitive, lacking response/underresponsivity, or seeking sensory input)
- Pattern 2: Sensory Discrimination Disorder, in which the individual has difficulty discriminating among stimuli (different modalities may be affected)
- Pattern 3: Sensory-Based Motor Disorder in which an individual's posture and muscle tone may be affected; the individual may have an inability to plan and execute motor action (Miller, Anzalone, Lane, Cermak, & Osten, 2007).

Figure 2.2 presents a schema of the proposed subtypes of SID/SPD. A review of the literature found that subtypes of SPD were discussed, with researchers concluding that more research is needed with comprehensive and consistent measures in children presenting with various disorders (Davies & Tucker, 2010). APNs should be aware that the understanding of SID/SPD is evolving as research further investigates this disorder within different clinical pictures.

Sensory issues have been found to be associated with prolonged institutional care in intercountry adopted children (Wilbarger, Gunnar,

Schneider, & Pollak, 2010). Children who had been in institutional care for greater than 12 months with more than 75% of their preadoption lives were compared with intercountry adopted children who had been cared for in foster care and with birth children. Children in institutional care had more significant difficulties in sensory modulation than the other groups (Wilbarger et al., 2010). APNs should also be aware that these sensory issues may extend to other social behaviors, such as emotions, posture, play, and attachment. Referral to occupational therapists may be helpful in diagnosing and managing sensory issues in adopted children.

EMOTIONAL/PSYCHOLOGICAL NEEDS

Attachment and Bonding

Psychologists and sociologists have articulated the interruption in attachment and bonding that some adopted and kinship children experience. Children who have experienced trauma, maltreatment, and chaotic home environments may show indiscriminate affection toward adults, lack empathy toward others, or have difficulty attaching to others. Adopted children's attachment (secure attachment versus disorganized attachment) was examined through meta-analyses (van den Dries, Juffer, van Ijzendoorn, & Bakermans-Kranenburg, 2009). The authors found that adopted children: (a) who were adopted after 1 year were less securely attached than nonadopted children; (b) overall had more disorganized attachments than nonadopted peers, but were comparable to foster care children; and (c) had less disorganized attachments than institutionalized children (van den Dries et al., 2009).

During the initial and subsequent follow-up with the child/adolescent and parent, the APN should observe parent–child and child–parent interactions to try to assess the status of attachment and bonding between the dyads. Asking caregivers what activities the child and they enjoy doing together may begin conversations related to attachment. Remember, this is reciprocal, and parents may be processing the child's needs within the family, which may have been challenging and disruptive. Referral to an adoption-informed mental health provider, for individual and family counseling, as well as respite care may be warranted.

Trauma

Imagine that your parents have been arrested and handcuffed, held at gunpoint by the sheriff's deputy—and you heard the sirens, the steps up to your porch, the loud knock on the door, and then the shouting of men's voices. Finally, you heard the cries and screams of your parents as they were put into the police car. Afterward, you were also taken to a new place to stay, a small suitcase or trash bag in hand with a few clothes and toys. And you were confused, hungry, and scared.

The child's experiences with traumatic events present an opportunity for APNs to apply their knowledge, skills, and attitudes with quality care in mind. The "Visit Discharge and Referral Summary for Family" form (AAP & Dave Thomas Foundation for Adoption, 2013) outlines documentation for trauma screening and current traumatic stress reactions, and can be located on the "Healthy Foster Care America: Primary Care Tools" website sponsored by the AAP. Being a trauma-informed provider is critical for diagnosing behaviors accurately. Understanding acute, chronic, complex, and developmental trauma will assist the APN in reaching differential diagnoses and an accurate plan of care. Traumatic events are discussed in further depth in Chapter 5.

Social and Spiritual Needs

Just as all of us do, individuals who were adopted travel through life trying to make sense of events and choices. For adopted persons and those under kinship care, there is more to their sense making: Why was I relinquished? Where did I come from? Who am I? Will I ever meet my birth mother and father? Am I destined to be the violent person my father was? Will I struggle with alcohol and drug use? Why do I resent my adoptive parents so much?

Discourse and language surrounding the adoption are especially important to allow these experiences to form meaning in a sacred manner. Tools such as creating "life books" tell the story of the adopted individual. Suggested rituals, such as those conducted on "Gotcha Days," the day the adopted child came to live with their "forever families," have been designed to assist adopted individuals create a personal narrative. Honoring the birth parents is considered crucial to the development of adopted and kinship children and adolescents. As one expert told me, "If the birth parent isn't honored, then how can you expect the adopted person to honor themselves?"

One influential author, Sherrie Eldridge, has transformed the conversations in popular culture for adopted persons. Her book series began with *Twenty Things Adopted Kids Wish Their Adoptive Parents Knew* (Eldridge, 1999) and has continued with several "twenty things" themes for adoptive parents and adopted persons. The common theme is to bring into the open conversations about how adopted persons view their world differently from those who are not adopted.

Disclosure of a child's adoption has grown beyond *whether* to disclose that the child was adopted. This was a question raised when physical matching and confidential adoptions were more commonplace. Now, it is about *how* and *when* the adoption is discussed between parents and their children. In a study conducted by Wydra, O'Brien, and Merson (2012), the majority of the conversations were positive; however, discomfort by the adoptive parents and withholding of information were also reported. Several parents had used books to facilitate disclosing that their child was adopted. How frequently adoption was discussed varied between families. Recommendations were to disclose adoption early in the child's life; the authors found that disclosures after age 5 were considered distressing to the adopted person (Wydra, O'Brien, & Merson, 2012). For conspicuous families, such as in transracial adoptions, conversations about adoption occur early in the child's life and may be an ongoing dialogue, depending upon the developmental stage and needs of the adopted person.

Kinship children also need to make sense of their pasts. The presence or absence of the birth parent may be both comforting and distressing, depending on circumstances. Regardless, the child may experience ambivalence and conflicting emotions because birth parents can simultaneously be both sources of trauma and individuals to whom the child is fiercely loyal.

MEDICALLY FRAGILE CHILDREN

Since the 1980s, there has been a marked increase in children born with complex medical needs, including HIV-positive infants and children.

Increasingly, children are born to drug- and alcohol-addicted mothers, often resulting in premature births and requiring complex neonatal care. We discuss therapeutic foster parents and children in foster care in Chapter 9. However, it should be noted here that foster parents do adopt children under their care, and not uncommonly, nurses will become therapeutic or special needs foster parents. For example, Angels in Waiting (n.d.) is a nonprofit agency created by nurses to care for the increasing population of medically fragile children in the foster care system in the United States (www.angelsinwaiting.org). Major cities, such as Chicago and New York, have societies devoted to caring for medically fragile children. The Department of Child Services (DCS) remains the guardian of these children as they are placed in therapeutic or medical foster care homes. Depending on the severity of the needs, visiting nurse services are included in the provision of care.

EDUCATION

Educating families and older children and adolescents should be performed with the goal of empowerment and facilitating ownership of health status to the family and child/adolescent. Ensuring safety, supporting capabilities, and providing emotional support during education are principles that will facilitate learning. Individualized education with understanding salient issues of the parents and child/adolescent are critical to ensure messages are delivered as effectively as possible. Protecting family members and preventing transmission of infectious diseases through universal precautions to understanding symptomatology based on chronic trauma are part of the wide range of education needed for adoptive and kinship families. The education plan should stem from assessment findings with an overall goal of optimizing individual and family functioning and adherence to the plan.

SUMMARY

As providers in primary and acute care settings, APNs render care to adopted and kinship children with optimal care delivered through medical homes. At times, APNs will be able to reach diagnoses and manage conditions; they will also need to suspend diagnoses and know when to collaborate and refer to specialists in adoption medicine, neurodevelopmental conditions, infectious diseases, psychologists/social workers, audiologists, occupational, speech/language, and physical therapists, and professionals in the education system. The role of the APN should not be minimized: APNs are providers who are well positioned to render holistic, informed care through gathering contextualized data and formulating a realistic, patient-centered plan of care.

CHAPTER HIGHLIGHTS

☐ Although the assessment and evaluation of adopted children/ adolescents should include the same parameters as those that apply to any pediatric patient, children in the care of adoptive and kinship parents are at risk for myriad physical, psychological, social, and learning challenges.

☐ APNs' assessments and plans of care will be guided by the past environments and current context of the infant/child. For adopted and kinship children, these contexts will be wide ranging, and APNs will need to appreciate the risk factors associated with these special pediatric groups of patients.

☐ APNs should be aware of the more common pediatric conditions that are amenable to management within their scope of practice and those requiring referral to a specialist. Providing patient-centered care and education through medical homes facilitates coordination of needed services.

Questions for Reflection

Following are a few questions to reflect upon. You can use these to start a journal for yourself or in a classroom discussion with peers and the instructor.

1. After reading this chapter, discuss what new insights you have regarding the evaluation of children in adoption and kinship families. What will you be sure to incorporate into your practice?

2. How do you view resiliency in children whose care has been suboptimal? Go to www.angelsinwaiting.org, and read the stories of infants who have overcome significant adversities. What role did nurses play in these children's lives?

3. How is holistic care for this group of children similar to and different from that for other children? What unique factors should be considered as the APN evaluates and plans care?
4. What research priorities do you assess after reading this chapter? What implications for policy?

References

AdoptUSKids. (2016). About us: Who we are. Retrieved from http://www.adoptuskids.org/about-us/who-we-are

Altarac, M., & Saroha, E. (2007). Lifetime prevalence of learning disability among U.S. children. *Pediatrics, 119*(Suppl. 1), S77–S83. doi:10.1542/peds.2006-2089L

American Academy of Pediatrics. (2005). *Fostering health: Health care for children and adolescents in foster care.* District II, NY: Author.

American Academy of Pediatrics. (2016a). AAP releases summary of updated preventive health care screening and assessment schedule for children's checkups. Retrieved from www.aap.org/en-us/about-the-aap/aap-press-room/pages/AAP-Releases-Summary-of-Updated-Preventive-Health-Care-Screening-and-Assessment-Schedule-for-Children's-Checkups.aspx?nfstatus=401&nftoken=00000000-0000-0000-0000-000000000000&nfstatusdescription=ERROR:+No+local+token

American Academy of Pediatrics. (2016b). *Healthy foster care America: Primary care tools.* Retrieved from www.aap.org/en-us/advocacy-and-policy/aap-health-initiatives/healthy-foster-care-america/Pages/Primary-Care-Tools.aspx?nfstatus=401&nftoken=00000000-0000-0000-0000-000000000000&nfstatusdescription=ERROR%3a+No+local+token#agingout

American Academy of Pediatrics (Committee on Infectious Diseases). (2015). *Red book: 2015 report of the committee on infectious diseases.* Elk Grove Village, IL: Author.

American Academy of Pediatrics (Section on Oral Health). (2014). Maintaining and improving on oral health of young children. *Pediatrics, 134*(6), 1224–1229. doi:10.1542/peds.2014-2984

American Academy of Pediatrics & Dave Thomas Foundation for Adoption. (2013). *Visit discharge and referral summary for family.* Retrieved from www.aap.org/en-us/advocacy-and-policy/aap-health-initiatives/healthy-foster-care-america/_layouts/15/WopiFrame.aspx?sourcedoc=/en-us/advocacy-and-policy/aap-health-initiatives/healthy-foster-care-america/Documents/DischargeForm.docx&action=default

American Psychiatric Association. (2013). *Diagnostic and statistical manual of mental disorders* (5th ed.). Arlington, VA: American Psychiatric Publishing.

American Speech-Language-Hearing Association. (2005). *(Central) auditory processing disorders* [Technical Report]. Retrieved from www.asha .org/policy/TR2005-00043

Angels in Waiting. (n.d.). Nursing clocking in at home & saving medically fragile foster care infants and children. Retrieved from angelsinwaiting.org

Autism Speaks®. (2016). *Autism speaks.* Retrieved from www.autismspeaks .org

Ayres, A. J. (1963). The development of perceptual-motor abilities: A theoretical basis for treatment dysfunction (Eleanor Clark Slagle Lecture). *American Journal of Occupational Therapy, 17,* 221–225.

Ayres, A. J. (1965). Patterns of perceptual-motor dysfunction in children: A factor analytic study. *Perceptual and Motor Skills, 20,* 335–368.

Bertrand, J., Floyd, R. L., Weber, M. K., O'Connor, M., Riley, E. P., Johnson, K. A.,... National Task Force on FAS/FAE. (2004). *Fetal alcohol syndrome: Guidelines for referral and diagnosis.* Atlanta, GA: Centers for Disease Control and Prevention.

Bramlett, M. D., Brooks, K. S., Foster, E. B., Satorius, J., Frasier, A. M., Skalland, B. J.,... Chowdhury, S. R. (2010). Design and operation of the National Survey of Adoptive Parents of Children with Special Health Care Needs, 2008. *Vital Health Stat, 1*(51), 1–118.

Bramlett, M. D., Radel, L. F., & Blumberg, S. J. (2007). The health and well-being of adopted children. *Pediatrics, 119,* S54–S60.

Centers for Disease Control and Prevention. (2015). Fetal alcohol spectrum disorders. Retrieved from www.cdc.gov/ncbddd/fasd/facts.html

Centers for Disease Control and Prevention. (2016). Autism and developmental disabilities monitoring (ADDM) network. Retrieved from www .cdc.gov/ncbddd/autism/addm.html

Chasnoff, I. J., Wells, A. M., & King, L. (2015). Misdiagnosis and missed diagnoses in foster and adopted children with prenatal alcohol exposure. *Pediatrics, 135*(2), 264–270. doi:10.1542/peds.2014-2171

Child Welfare Information Gateway. (2016). *Foster care statistics 2014.* Washington, DC: U.S. Department of Health and Human Services, Children's Bureau.

Clark, M. B., Slayton, R. L., & Section on Oral Health. (2014). Fluoride use in caries prevention in the primary care setting. *Pediatrics, 134*(3), 626–633. doi:10.1542/peds.2014-1699

Coles, C. (2014). Prenatal substance exposure: Alcohol and other substances—Implications for adoption. In P. W. Mason, D. E. Johnson, & L. A. Prock (Eds.), *Adoption medicine: Caring for children and families* (pp. 97–122). Elk Grove Village, IL: American Academy of Pediatrics.

Council on Foster Care, Adoption and Kinship Care, Committee on Adolescence, & Council on Early Childhood. (2015). Health care issues for children and adolescents in foster care and kinship care. *Pediatrics, 136*(4), e1131–e1140. doi:10.1542/peds.2015-2655

Crea, T. M., Chan, K., & Barth, R. P. (2013). Family environment and attention-deficit/hyperactivity disorder in adopted children: Associations with family cohesion and adaptability. *Child: Care, Health and Development, 40*(6), 853–862. doi:10.1111/cch.12112

Damsteegt, R. C., van IJzendoom, M. H., Out, D., & Bakermans-Kranenburg, M. J. (2014). Tympanic membrane temperature in adopted children associated with sleep problems and pre-adoption living arrangements: An exploratory study. *BMC Psychology, 2*(1), 51. doi:10.1186/s40359-014-0051-2

Davies, P. L., & Tucker, R. (2010). Evidence review to investigate the support for subtypes of children with difficulty processing and integrating sensory information. *American Journal of Occupational Therapy, 64*(3), 391–402. doi:10.5014/ajot.2010.09070

Doom, J. R., Gunnar, M. R., Georgieff, M. K., Kroupina, M. G., Frenn, K., Fuglestad, A. J., Carlson, S. M. (2014). Beyond stimulus deprivation: Iron deficiency and cognitive deficits in postinstitutionalized children. *Child Development, 85*(3), 1805–1812. doi:10.1111/cdev.12231

Eldridge, S. (1999). *Twenty things adopted kids wish their adoptive parents knew.* New York, NY: Dell Publishing.

Ezell, J., Shui, A., Sanders, K., & Veenstra-VanderWeele, J. (2016). Pattern of diagnosis and co-occurring symptoms in adopted children with autism spectrum disorder. *Pediatrics, 137*(S2):S90–S97. doi:10.1542peds2015-2851G

Finnegan, L. P., Connaughton J. F., Jr., Kron, R. E., & Emich, J. P. (1975). Neonatal abstinence syndrome: Assessment and management. *Additive Diseases, 2*(1-2), 141–158.

Flak, A. L., Su, S., Bertrand, J., Denny, C. H., Kresmodel, U. S., & Cogswell, M. E. (2014). The association of mild, moderate, and binge prenatal alcohol exposure and child neuropsychological outcomes: A meta-analysis. *Alcoholism: Clinical and Experimental Research, 38*(1), 214–226. doi:10.1111/acer.12214

Frankenburg, W. K., Dodds, J., Archer, P., Shapiro, H., & Bresnick, B. (1992). The DENVER II: A major revision and restandardization of the Denver Developmental Screening Test. *Pediatrics, 89*(1), 91–97.

Fuglestad, A. J., Georgieff, M. K., Iverson, S. L., Miller, B. S., Petryk, A., Johnson, D. E., & Kroupina, M. G. (2013). Iron deficiency after arrival is associated with general cognitive and behavioral impairment in post-institutionalized children adopted from Eastern Europe. *Maternal and Child Health Journal, 17*, 1080–1087. doi:10.1007/s10995-012-1090-z

Hayward, R. A., DePanfilis, D., & Woodruff, K. (2010). Parental methamphetamine use and implications for child welfare intervention: A review of the literature. *Journal of Public Child Welfare, 4*(1), 25–60. doi:10.1080/15548730903563095

Jansson, L. M., Velez, M., & Harrow, C. (2009). The opioid-exposed newborn: Assessment and pharmacologic management. *Journal of Opioid Management, 5*(1), 47–55.

Johnson, C. P., & Myers, S. (2007). Identification and evaluation of children with autism spectrum disorders. *Pediatrics, 120*(5), 1183–1215. doi:10.1542/peds.2007-2361

Jones, V. F., & Committee on Early Childhood, Adoption and Dependent Care (High, P. C., Donoghue, E., Fussell, J. J., Gleason, M. M., Jaudes, P. K., Rubin, D. M., & Schulte, E.). (2012). Comprehensive health evaluation of the newly adopted child. *Pediatrics, 129*(1), e214–e223. doi:10.1542/peds.2011-2381

Jones, H. E., & Fielder, A. (2015). Neonatal abstinence syndrome: Historical perspective, current focus, future directions. *Preventive Medicine. 80*, 12–17. doi:10.1016/j.ypmed.2015.07.017

Juffer, F., & van IJzendoorn M. H. (2005). Behavior problems and mental health referrals of international adoptees: A meta-analysis. *Journal of the American Medical Association, 293*, 2501–2515.

Kim, J., & Staat, M. A. (2004). Acute care issues in internationally adopted children. *Clinical Pediatric Emergency Medicine, 5*(2), 130–142. doi:10.1016/j.cpem.2004.01.005

Krandall, S. R., & Gartner, L. M. (1974). Late presentation of drug withdrawal symptoms in newborns. *American Journal of Diseases of Children, 127*, 58–61.

Kranowitz, C. S. (2005). *The out-of-sync child.* New York, NY: Berkley Publishing Group.

Kuczmarski, R. J., Ogden, C. L., Guo, S. S., Grummer-Strawn, L. M., Flegal, K. M., Mei, Z., . . . Johnson, C. L. (2002). 2000 CDC growth charts for the United States: Methods and development. *Vital Health Statistics 11*, (246), 1–192.

Learning Disabilities Navigator. (2013a). Introduction. Retrieved from http://ldnavigator.ncld.org/#/intro/learning-disabilities/5

Learning Disabilities Navigator. (2013b). Learning disabilities defined. Retrieved from http:// ldnavigator.ncld.org/#/ld-defined/bridging -the-divide/1

Mason, P. W., Johnson, D. E., & Prock, L. A. (Eds.). (2014). *Adoption medicine*. Elk Grove Village, IL: American Academy of Pediatrics.

McGuinness, T. M., & Pollack, D. (2008). Parental methamphetamine abuse and children. *Journal of Pediatric Health Care, 22*(3), 152–158. doi:10.1016/j .pedhc.2007.04.009

Miller, L. J., Anzalone, M. E., Lane, S. J., Cermak, S. A., & Osten, E. T. (2007). Concept evolution in sensory integration: A proposed nosology for diagnosis. *American Journal of Occupational Therapy, 61*(2), 135–140.

National Center for Learning Disabilities. (2016). The LD navigator by ld.org. Retrieved from ldnavigator.ncld.org

National Center on Substance Abuse and Child Welfare. (n.d.). Fact sheet 3—Research studies on the prevalence of substance use disorders in the child welfare population. Retrieved from www.ncsacw.samhsa.gov /files/Research_Studies_Prevalence_Factsheets.pdf

Rakhlin, N., Hein, S., Doyle, N., Hart, L., Macomber, D., Ruchkin, V.,... Grigorenko, E. L. (2015). Language development of internationally adopted children: Adverse early experiences outweigh the age of acquisition effect. *Journal of Communication Disorders, 57*, 66–80. doi:10.1016/j .jcomdis.2015.08.003

Rettig, M., & McCarthy-Rettig, K. (2006). A survey of the health, sleep, and development of children adopted from China. *Health & Social Work, 31*(3), 201–207.

Robins, D. L., Casagrande, K., Barton, M., Chen, C. A., Dumont-Mathieu, T., & Fein, D. (2014). Validation of the modified checklist for autism in toddlers, revised with follow-up (M-CHAT-R/F). *Pediatrics, 133*(1), 37–45. doi:10.1542/peds.2013-1813

Robins, D. L., Fein, D., & Barton, M. (2009). *The Modified Checklist for Autism in Toddlers, Revised with Follow-Up (M-CHAT-R/F)*. Self-published.

Schulte, E. E., & Springer, S. H. (2014). Post-adoptive evaluation for health care professionals. In P. W. Mason, D. E. Johnson, & L. A. Prock (Eds.), *Adoption medicine: Caring for Children and Families* (pp. 163–175). Elk Grove Village, IL: American Academy of Pediatrics.

Simmel, C., Brooks, D., Barth, R. P., & Hinshaw, S. P. (2001). Externalizing symptomatology among adoptive youth: Prevalence and preadoption risk factors. *Journal of Abnormal Child Psychology, 29*(1), 57–69.

Smith, S. L. (2010). Keeping the promise: The critical need for post-adoption services to enable children and families to succeed. New York, NY: Donaldson Adoption Institute. Retrieved from http://adoptioninstitute .org/research/2010_10_promises.php

Smith, S. L. (2013). A family for life: The vital need to achieve permanency for children in care. New York, NY: Donaldson Adoption Institute. Retrieved from http://adoptioninstitute.org/research/2013_04_Family ForLife.php

Smith, S. L. (2014). *Supporting and preserving adoptive families: Profiles of publicly funded post-adoption services.* New York, NY: The Donaldson Institute.

van den Dries, L., Juffer, F., van Ijzendoorn, M. H., & Bakermans-Kranenburg, M. J. (2009). Fostering security? A meta-analysis of attachment in adopted children. *Children and Youth Services Review, 31*, 410–421. doi:10.1016/j.childyouth.2008.09.008

Vandivere, S., Malm, K., & Radel, L. (2009). *Adoption USA: A chartbook based on the 2007 National Survey of Adoptive Parents.* Washington, DC: The U.S. Department of Health and Human Services, Office of the Assistant Secretary for Planning and Evaluation.

World Health Organization, Multicentre Growth Reference Study Group. (2006). *WHO Child Growth Standards: Length/height-for-age, weight-for-age, weight-for-length, weight-for-height and body mass index-for-age: Methods and development.* Geneva, Switzerland: World Health Organization.

Wilbarger, J., Gunnar, M., Schneider, M., & Pollak, S. (2010). Sensory processing in internationally adopted, post-institutionalized children. *The Journal of Child Psychology and Psychiatry, 51*(10), 1105–1114. doi:10.1111/j.1469-7610.2010.02255.x

Wydra, M., O'Brien, K. M., & Merson, E. S. (2012). In their own words: Adopted persons' experiences of adoption disclosure and discussion in their families. *Journal of Family Social Work, 15*(1), 62–77. doi:10.1080/1052 2158.2012.642616

3

Birth Parents

□ □ □ □

PURPOSE OF THE CHAPTER

In this chapter, we discuss what it iEs to be a birth parent who relinquishes a child through the formal adoption process. Singularly unique as members of the adoption triad, birth parents' legal, gendered, political, financial, and emotional rights have been the theme of books, movies, and, more recently, social media. The struggle to make the decision to create an adoption plan is never an easy one, but it must be one that is made with full informed consent and disclosure. Issues of the rights of minors (when birth parents are under 18 years of age), as well as those of class and race come into focus as we examine birth parents' decisions to relinquish a child. Some would argue that adoption is merely the commodification of children, with the elite class (adoptive parents) benefiting from those who are less fortunate with fewer resources and opportunities. Indeed, birth mothers are found in high school (and later, having dropped out of high school), the "working poor," and in developing countries across the globe.

We also briefly explore the experience of those parents who do not voluntarily release parental rights of their children and how relinquishment affected them long after placement. In our case studies, stories are presented of a 65-year-old birth father who has recently discovered that he has a daughter, a teenager faced with an unexpected pregnancy, a couple whose vulnerable economic situation and fragile relationship make parenting a child difficult, and a birth mother experiencing grief and postpartum depression (PPD) after relinquishing a baby. We explore these members of the adoption triad and place the important role of the advanced practice nurse (APN) within social and health care contexts.

Learning Objectives

At the completion of the chapter, the reader will be able to:

1. Identify the various contexts in which parents may voluntarily or involuntarily relinquish parental rights
2. Discuss the heterogeneity of birth parents, which influences their motivations to create an adoption plan
3. Define open/closed adoptions, including implications for the birth parents
4. Examine policies and government initiatives related to birth parents, including Safe Haven Laws and the Infant Adoption Awareness Training Program
5. Analyze methods to assess for substance use in pregnant women with an awareness of state laws that require reporting of substance use
6. Identify the signs and symptoms of disenfranchised grief of a birth mother and father who have relinquished their infant in the peripartum setting

RELINQUISHMENT OF A CHILD

Domestic Adoption

Today, there are fewer infants available for private adoption, with demand outpacing supply. If this sounds like an economic principle, it is. And there are multiple and vocal critiques of domestic private adoption, criticisms that are based on the perception of commodification of human life. Perhaps more than any other triad member, birth parents often come with an emotional component that cascades from experiences of loss, difficult choices, and issues of class and gender. More recently, with the onset of "open adoptions," such experiences have been mitigated or, at least, addressed at some level. Birth parents have been depicted as victims of forced relinquishment (e.g., *The Lost Child of Philomena Lee* by journalist Martin Sixsmith), and their own genre of birth parent narratives has been created. Indeed, parental rights may be voluntarily or involuntarily terminated, as described in Chapter 1.

Unintended Pregnancies

In 2008, unintended pregnancies accounted for 51% of all pregnancies; 54 per 1,000 women ages 15 to 44 years of age experienced an unintended pregnancy resulting in 27 per 1,000 births (Finer & Zolna, 2014). What is also of note is that there were large disparities in relationship status, income, and education, disparities that have increased over time (between 2001 and 2008). The number of unintended pregnancies ending in abortion decreased and that of births increased. Racial disparities revealed that Black women had the highest rates of unintended pregnancies, with Hispanic women having the highest rates of births resulting from unintended pregnancies (Finer & Zolna, 2014). Women are choosing to raise their children because the pressure of social mores on single mothers to relinquish their children has greatly diminished.

Termination of Parental Rights

In cases of involuntary termination of parental rights, mental health issues or maltreatment of the child is evident, either as neglect or abuse. A plan will be created for parents to follow in order to "get their kids back" and may include negative drug screens. Adherence to the plan will determine whether the child is ultimately available to be adopted. If the plan is not followed or if other circumstances are present that impair individuals from parenting the child, the court terminates such rights, and allows the child to then be available for placement through the foster care system. The time for this process varies with families and situations.

When rights are terminated, birth parents have little to no voice in who will be the next caregivers of their children. In effect, they have lost that right and often blame the foster parents who step in to care for their children. Feelings of anger and powerlessness are often voiced. Informed foster parents will understand that, when possible, creating a partnership with the birth parent supports acting in the child's interests.

On the other hand, in private domestic adoption, birth parents have the ability to select adoptive parents from profiles posted online and through adoption agencies and attorneys. They can view the narratives written by prospective parents, which often describe religious background, professions, other children in the home, and sexual orientation. Birth parents can, on the basis of this information, select those individuals to whom they would like to release their child.

Regardless, many vocal critics of adoption believe that there is little choice for birth parents who relinquish a child. Economic hardship creates a "no-win" scenario for those who decide to create an adoption plan. The word "choice," some would argue, is not accurate. Others disagree and have made a plan they know is the right path for them. The desire to parent may not be part of their desired life experiences, and they have selected individuals who very much want a child in their lives. For APNs, approaching birth parents in an open, respectful manner is important. Understand that individual narratives will differ and that parents' emotional paradigms toward relinquishment present in vastly different ways. The APN must allow each birth parent to have a voice.

Expenses During Pregnancy

After private domestic birth parents select prospective adoptive parents, certain expenses are allowable, which cannot be viewed as coercive. As with so many laws overseeing adoption, state statutes show some variation in what is considered allowable, as well as the time the expenses are allowed after placement (30 days to 6 months). Allowable expenses typically include maternity-related health care costs, temporary living expenses of the mother during pregnancy, psychological counseling fees, legal fees, and travel fees related to the adoption (Child Welfare Information Gateway, 2013a). Payment that is in any way construed as "baby selling," is strictly prohibited. The APN assesses for coercive influencing of a birth parent who plans to place the infant through domestic private adoption through payment of expenses or in other ways.

Labor, Delivery, and Postpartum Issues

Being with a birth parent at the time of delivering a baby who is being relinquished can evoke emotions within the health care professional. The paradox of loss and joy is pronounced. Hospital policies are followed, usually with the social worker taking the lead in the process. "BUFA" is sometimes used as a term to indicate "baby up for adoption"; however, many hospitals are no longer using this language, which some find offensive—the acronym is confusing, and the baby is a person with a name. However, this acronym symbolizes the transitional period when the child is being released into the care of new parents, who may rename the baby.

Health care organizations' policies will often stipulate that staff are to remain neutral, not persuading or dissuading a parent's decision related to the adoption. Often, however, the birth mother's grief and at times revisiting the decision to relinquish the baby will evoke emotions within the nurse who is caring for the mother. Adoptive parents have described to me how, at times, nurses, although not influencing the birth mother's decision, have held undeserved negative attitudes toward them. Nurses may believe the birth mother is being taken advantage of, and witnessing the intense emotions of grief, loss, and sadness is difficult. There are a few guiding principles to remember in this scenario. First, separate the birth parents' decision to relinquish a child from the placement of the child to the adoptive parents. Avoid a "bad guy/good guy" judgment. No birth parent should ever be coerced into placing a child (unless parental rights have been terminated due to maltreatment, which has been decided by the courts). Regardless, such relinquishment should not create negative feelings toward the adoptive parents. Second, a personal inventory of emotions may be helpful. Depending on your personal story, such situations may be a personal trauma reminder. Be aware that the compassion you feel toward the birth mother may interfere with your understanding that the adoptive parent also needs your care.

Social service staff members are often the primary professionals to coordinate the adoption events: the signature of adoption consent papers and the timing of them, and the completion of forms for caring for the infant. Court documents may be separate from the medical record; state law will dictate privacy of the parent and child, sealing of the original birth certificate, and whether medical information is de-identified. The secrecy surrounding adoption has begun.

Despite the social worker orchestrating the events postbirth, the nurse also has significant influence over how these delicate, fragile interactions are remembered and how meaning attributed to this life event commences. What do you say to a weeping birth mother as she hands her child to the adoptive mother? How do you react when no one else is looking and you see the grief covering the birth parent's face? How do you interpret contentment from a birth mother who has thoughtfully and carefully created this plan? When the decision to relinquish is rescinded, what do you say to remain neutral?

In my study that surveyed nurses who cared for the adoption triad, three major areas of concern were reported by nurses who cared for birth parents: emotional health (resolving and healing); relinquishment decision making (Was this the right choice?); and adoption issues (What happens after my child is placed?; Foli, 2012). The fear of being judged, concerns about the adoptive parents, and conflict with family members over the decision to place the baby were described (Foli, 2012). In this study, nurses were asked what interventions were most effective for birth parents during this time. Psychosocial support, therapeutic communication, follow-up services and referrals, and advocacy were the major areas described. Nurses need to ensure policy is followed by advocating that the birth parents' rights are upheld throughout the process, including care of the baby. Ultimately, it is the comfort, health status (postoperative recovery from cesarean section to drug/alcohol withdrawal), and preferences of birth parents that supersede others during the time during which the adoption plan is carried out (see Exhibit 3.1).

EXHIBIT 3.1

BIRTH PARENT ISSUES AND CONCERNS AND NURSING INTERVENTIONS

Concerns

Emotional health: Resolving and healing
- ☐ *Guilt*
- ☐ *Depression*
- ☐ *Grief/loss*
- ☐ *Trauma/trauma of separation*
- ☐ *Fear of being judged/ "I am not a bad person"*
- ☐ *Stoic behavior/avoid baby*
- ☐ *Stress*
- ☐ *Anger*
- ☐ *Drug/ethanol*

(continued)

EXHIBIT 3.1 *(continued)*

Relinquishment decision making: Was this the right choice?
☐ Uncertainty/Is adoption the right choice?
☐ Influence from family members who disagree with adoption plan
☐ Changing the adoption decision

Adoption issues: What happens after the child is placed?
☐ Concern regarding adoptive home
☐ Society's judgment
☐ Inadequate pre-/postadoption counseling/lack of support
☐ Not knowing about the child or adoptive parents not keeping in contact as they had promised
☐ Adoptive parents involved in birth experience

Nursing Interventions

Psychosocial support
☐ Understand conflicted feelings
☐ Grief counseling
☐ Reassure decision/choice was appropriate
☐ Self-esteem: "not a bad person"
☐ Acceptance/validation/affirmation/respect
☐ Nurse: Be willing to talk with birth parents

Therapeutic communication
☐ Active listening
☐ Nonjudgmental approach

Follow-up services/referrals
☐ Social worker (when child leaves hospital)
☐ Counselor

Advocacy
☐ Understand rights
☐ Lack of pressure to relinquish
☐ Involvement with care of child

Source: Foli (2012).

The presence of adoptive parents—often seen as obtrusive and invading privacy—is another factor of which nurses need to be aware. Often, especially when open adoption arrangements have been negotiated, adoptive parents will attend prenatal checkups and be present in the labor and delivery room with the birth mother/father. Many nurses and physicians may not understand such arrangements and think it "unusual" and even "unnatural" for such parties to attend these intimate moments. Yet others view it as the integration of two families with the ultimate goal of supporting both the child's well-being and the birth parents' lifelong tie with the child.

Intercountry Adoption

Often, relinquishment of an infant or child in developing nations is based on several factors, including economic hardship, stigma of out-of-wedlock pregnancies, and gender bias, with infant girls being relinquished more than boys. In select countries, there is now a lopsided gender distribution and other factors, such as higher rates of abortion for female fetuses that have caused concern in these countries. In 1978, the Chinese government instituted the one-child campaign in response to concerns over population growth. Couples were to stop procreating after one child, regardless of gender. Thus, the rule was "bound to lead to difficulties given the immense symbolic and practical importance of male offspring within Chinese society" (Wasserstrom, 1984, pp. 346–347). As a result of this, female infanticide was found, especially in rural areas, and more female babies were relinquished for intercountry adoption. This gender bias was not isolated to China. Roberts and Montgomery (2016) presented an alarming analysis of the disproportionate gender distribution in a rural mission hospital in India. Using data from the hospital and comparing gender birth rates with state ratios, the authors found hospital female-to-male ratios lower than state gender ratios. Further, qualitative themes derived from 17 interviews with women were social norms and expectations of fertility, preference for male children, and health-related decision making, which may be associated with aborting female fetuses. The strong bias toward male offspring, with roots in both culture and finances (dowry costs of females), was attributed to this disproportionate ratio (Roberts & Montgomery, 2016). Besides more females being released for adoption, special needs infants are also relinquished through intercountry adoption. Today, many adoption agencies have rigorous in-country placement programs so that infants and children are adopted within their countries whenever possible.

In intercountry adoptions, accounts of infants being taken from unsuspecting birth parents in developing countries prompted the passing of the Hague Convention (see Chapter 1). Eliminating third parties who have financial interests in arranging for adoptions was one of the goals of this treaty. However, others argue that the Hague Convention needs to enforce stiffer penalties on those who duplicitously take children away from unsuspecting birth parents who are misled into signing away their rights (Manley, 2006).

Although reunions with birth parents from other countries have been uncommon, many parents and their children are seeking to find lost family members. Individuals who were adopted from Korea, China, Haiti, Russia, and Vietnam are seeking—and at times finding—their birth families. The popular press offers descriptions of adult children who have found birth parents in countries outside the United States.

Safe Haven Laws

There are instances when no adoption plan—or any plan to care for the child—is made. A significant crisis envelops birth parents, making them feel they have nowhere to turn. Keeping such grave instances in view, the National Safe Haven Laws (see Exhibit 3.2) were designed to protect infants from abandonment and their parents from prosecution, *if the baby is left safely at a Safe Haven location*. These extreme situations affect APNs working in acute care facilities as well as community-based organizations. The infant who has been left via a Safe Haven Law needs to be assessed immediately and when stable, turned over to child protection services to be placed with a foster family.

EXHIBIT 3.2
SAFE HAVEN LAWS

The Safe Haven Laws, also called "Baby Moses laws," are instituted in all 50 states, the District of Columbia, and Puerto Rico. These laws are designed to protect infants from unsafe abandonment. However, state laws differ. For example, the age of the infant at the time of relinquishment differs between states. The question of who may relinquish the infant also varies by state (e.g., either custodial parent or someone with legal custody of the child). Finally, the question of what party the infant is relinquished to is determined differently in many states. Safe Haven locations in some states require that the infant be given to a hospital or health care facility; others allow police stations and churches. Parental rights may be terminated immediately or, as in some states, after a waiting period. Regardless, these laws serve to provide birth parents with anonymity and protection from criminal prosecution for abandonment.

The National Safe Haven Alliance (www.nationalsafehav-enalliance.org) is a not-for-profit organization that supports Safe Haven laws and seeks to prevent harm to abandoned infants. They have established a Safe Haven Confidential Crisis Hotline: 1-888-510-BABY (2229).

Safety of the Unborn Child and Mother

The APN is also responsible for assessing for alcohol and substance abuse during the birth mother's pregnancy. However, ethical questions may cloud decisions in the provision of care. For example, state mandatory screening and reporting guidelines may conflict with values against treating the patient as a criminal. The APN's care will be guided by whether the patient is viewed as an individual who breaks the law or as an individual with a disease state that is jeopardizing her life and the life of her unborn child, as well as mandatory reporting and referral guidance in the state of practice.

The surge in abuse of opioids has spurred several health care organizations to forward policy statements so that providers are guided in the delivery of compassionate and safe care. The Association of Women's Health, Obstetric, and Neonatal Nurses (AWHONN; 2015) has issued a position statement:

> [AWHONN] opposes laws and other reporting requirements that result in incarceration or other punitive legal actions against women because of a substance abuse disorder in pregnancy. (p. 155)

The statement goes on to add, however, that nurses should be familiar with state laws on mandatory reporting and referrals, and follow these laws. Further, the organization supports universal screening for substance use in pregnant women. AWHONN views addiction as a disease, not as a criminal act (AWHONN, 2015). Similarly, the American Congress of Obstetricians and Gynecologists (ACOG, n.d., 2011/2014) emphasizes that evidence does not support the threat of or incarceration of pregnant women in deterring substance abuse. Rather, targeted treatment is encouraged and includes safe prescribing authority for opioid-agonist therapy (OAT; ACOG, n.d.). ACOG summarizes major points in "Actions to Support Healthy Outcomes for Mom and Baby" (see Table 3.1).

APN Screening and Management of Substance Use

Although a detailed explanation of treatment of substance use is beyond the purpose of this guide, the SBIRT approach (Screening, Brief Intervention, Brief Therapy, and Referral to Treatment) is an evidence-based practice supported by the Substance Abuse and Mental Health Services Administration (SAMHSA). In 2003, the federal government established the SBIRT grantee program through SAMHSA; data from grantees support the effectiveness of the program (i.e., reduction in alcohol and drug use; improvement in quality of life measures; and reduction in risky behaviors; Office of National Drug Control Policy & Substance Abuse and Mental Health Services Administration, 2012).

Screening questions will identify those who are using substances in a high-risk or unhealthy way; most patients will screen negative.

TABLE 3.1 *Actions to Support Healthy Outcomes for Mom and Baby*

Does Not Support Healthy Outcomes for Mom and Baby	Supports Healthy Outcomes for Mom and Baby
Overtreatment of NAS in NICUs	Appropriate comfort care in low-stimuli environment and pharmacological therapy where indicated
Criminal penalties for women and doctors	Public health approaches focused on prevention and treatment
Mandatory urine testing	Screening dialogue/questionnaire with patient consent
Mandatory reporting to law enforcement or child protective services (CPS)	Statistical reporting to department of health or direct reporting to CPS only for indications of impaired parenting
Overreliance on fragmented PDMPs	Safe prescribing and initial check of PDMPs
Punitive drug treatment courts	Family-centered drug treatment programs
Restrictions on medication access and forced withdrawal	OAT with methadone or buprenorphine for women and protections for treating physicians
Misleading drug prescribing warnings	Evidence-based labeling of opioid medications
Antifamily, one-size-fits-all drug treatment programs	Family-centered, community-based, outpatient treatment
Coercive referrals for fertility control	Counseling on pregnancy, planning, prevention, and contraception
Losing sight of the real harms of alcohol and cigarette use during pregnancy	Continued focus on the greatest preventable health threats—alcohol and tobacco use during pregnancy

NAS, Neonatal Abstinence Syndrome; NICU, neonatal intensive care unit; OAT, opioid agonist therapy; PDMPs, prescription drug monitoring programs.

Source: American Congress of Obstetricians and Gynecologists (n.d.).

Brief Interventions and Brief Therapy are designed to provide feedback and education and instill insight by use of strategic interviewing techniques. Referral to Treatment is the last step and is used for individuals for whom substance use disorders require further assessment and/or treatment. This approach is used for individuals who present with unhealthy or risky consumption of substances, or who may need to be further evaluated for substance use disorders (Exhibit 3.3). Codes for reimbursable SBIRT services are also of note, including commercial insurance, Medicare, and Medicaid.

The skilled APN will be able to use the principles of SBIRT when assessing pregnant women, beginning with screening for alcohol, tobacco, and drug use.

EXHIBIT 3.3

SBIRT Approach: Four Steps

SBIRT at a Glance

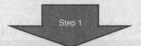

Step 1

Screen Patients
Screening quickly assesses the severity of substance use and identifies the appropriate level of treatment. Screenings take place in trauma centers, emergency rooms, community clinics, health centers, dental clinics, and school clinics. Screening can be done through one to five pre-screen questions based on evidence from NIDA and NIAAA.

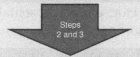

Steps 2 and 3

Conduct Brief Intervention and Brief Therapy
Brief Intervention and Brief Therapy use motivational interviewing techniques to increase a person's awareness of substance use and encourage changes in behavior.

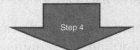

Step 4

Refer to Treatment
Referral to treatment offers access to specialty care for individuals who are in need of treatment for substance abuse.

NIAAA, National Institute of Alcohol Abuse and Alcoholism; NIDA, National Institute on Drug Abuse.
Source: Office of National Drug Control Policy & Substance Abuse and Mental Health Services Administration (2012).

Another online resource, also sponsored by SAMHSA, is the Providers' Clinical Support System for Opioid Therapy (PCSS-O): "a national training and mentoring project developed in response to the prescription opioid overdose epidemic" (Providers' Clinical Support System for Opioid Therapy, n.d.). Developed by physicians and APNs, this online resource contains training modules, webinars, and mentoring support for providers in the treatment of opioid dependence. Informed APNs, combined with early screening and intervention, will contribute to outcomes such as healthier pregnancies and fewer complications from alcohol and drug use.

ADOPTION PLAN

In the majority of child relinquishment situations, the birth parents have time to consider their options, despite very often feeling that they are in crisis. Representatives and legislators in Congress appear to be invested in ensuring that birth parents are presented with all options when faced with an unexpected pregnancy: raising the child, terminating the pregnancy, *and* adoption (see Infant Adoption Awareness Training Program later in this chapter). The 114th Congress has introduced a bill in the House of Representatives, H.R. 3428, called the Adoption Information Act (Congress.gov, 2016):

> [The Act] amends the Public Health Service Act to require family planning service projects or programs, as a condition of receiving certain grants or contracts, to assure the Secretary of Health and Human Services (HHS) that they will provide each person who inquires about their services with a pamphlet containing a comprehensive list of adoption centers in their state.

If passed, this Bill would require funded agencies to give specific information related to adoption as a requirement for continued federal support. Overall, however, little research has been conducted on how women choose adoption as a reproductive choice. In a study conducted by Sisson (2015), 40 women who had placed an infant for adoption between 1962 and 2009 were interviewed. Contrary to popular assumptions, most birth mothers who relinquished a child did not see their choice as being between adoption and abortion; rather it was between adoption and parenting the child. Most of the mothers who had a positive experience with adoption were in open adoption situations, and whether the adoption was open or closed was the biggest predictor of adoption satisfaction (Sisson, 2015).

When minors become pregnant, the issue of consent for placing the baby becomes even more complex because issues of full disclosure, developmental age, and potential for coercion surface. As with so many aspects of adoption law, states vary widely with regard to the minor birth mother's legal rights. Twenty-eight states and the District of Columbia allow minors to release their children to adoption independently. In contrast, five states require parental involvement, and five states require legal counsel. Finally, 12 states have no legal guidance or policy when a minor becomes pregnant and chooses to create an adoption plan (Guttmacher Institute, 2016). When presented with a minor who is pregnant and considering an adoption plan, the APN should consult state laws to determine the birth mother's legal rights.

Openness in Adoption

An important component of the adoption plan is how much contact or openness will be arranged between the birth and adoptive parents. As reviewed in the history of adoption and mentioned in the study by Sisson (2015) cited previously, varying levels of openness in adoptions have become normative, depending upon the time period. Postadoption connections between birth and adoptive parents exist on a continuum from closed or confidential, to semi-open or mediated, to open with face-to-face visits between birth and adoptive families (see Figure 3.1). In essence, open adoption allows some form of contact between birth parents and the child. Since the mid- to late 1980s, open adoptions have been increasingly common and viewed as being in the best interest of the child (Siegel & Smith, 2012; Wolfgram, 2008).

Evidence supports positive outcomes with open adoption. Siegel (2012) reported that young adults who had been adopted and were part of an open adoption described the dynamics as opportunities to develop identity, expand family, and process feelings. More studies are needed to verify the empirical evidence collected thus far. As in many instances of evidence-based practices, individual needs and circumstances should be fully evaluated. For example, in the

FIGURE 3.1   *Continuum of contact between birth and adoptive parents.*
Source: Child Welfare Information Gateway (2013c).

Confidential Adoption	Semi-Open Adoption (Mediated)	Open Adoption
• No contact	• Indirect contact	• Direct communication
• No identifying information shared	• Share nonidentifying information	• Exchange identifying information

instances of involuntary termination of parental rights, particularly with parental chronic substance abuse disorders, a history of family violence, or maltreatment of the child, open adoption arrangements need to be carefully considered in light of child safety.

Furthermore, when investigating open adoption agreements, birth parents should be advised that postadoption contact agreements vary in the ability to legally enforce them. Postadoption contact agreement laws between birth and adoptive families differ from state to state (to find specific state laws, see: www.childwelfare.gov/systemwide/laws_policies/state/). Many birth parents request postadoption contact as a condition of adoption; however, some prefer to have a closed adoption. Having contact with birth parents gives adopted persons a link to their past as well as access to genetic and medical information. APNs should be aware that there are factors to open adoption contracts that may be difficult at times for all parties. Social workers admit that, at times, there are more complexities with open agreements, but that the effort is worthwhile. The welfare of the child and the long-term benefits should be weighed on an individual basis (Child Welfare Information Gateway, 2013c).

Birth Fathers

Biologically, the woman's body changes as the pregnancy progresses, and it becomes obvious to society that a child is growing within her. In contrast, the man undergoes no such physical changes and can blend into society without communicating his parentage. The "double standard" in sexual behaviors also contributes to the perceptions that fathers do not experience the same emotional consequences as birth mothers do within the context of adoption. But I am not convinced these assumptions are accurate. I spoke to an adoptive family whose child (while in foster care) needed a medical procedure. The birth father had been notified about the procedure, but no one expected him to come. However, he did come and was given the opportunity to relay just how much the child meant to him and how marginalized he had felt. Yet historically, birth fathers have been given little to no voice in the placement of their children. Reflecting these practices, an historical document published by the Child Welfare League of America (1960) stated:

> Within the United States, the unmarried mother has sole rights to custody of her child. . . . The unmarried father has *no* legal right to the custody of his child. He has only a moral obligation to support, unless he has formally acknowledged paternity or legal adjudication of paternity has been made through court action. In such cases, in many states the father does not acquire the legal status of a parent and his consent to wardship or adoption is not required. However, if adoption is planned, an agency should safeguard the child and itself against future litigation by obtaining consent, waiver or disclaimer whenever possible, even when there has been only informal admission of paternity. (p. 17)

This document, more than half a century old, reaches into modern society, which views the father as a secondary parent, even reflected in hospitals' policies and procedures during the relinquishment process (where their absence is surely notable). Thus, some individuals would argue that birth fathers are not given their due voice in the adoption decision–making process. The media case of "Baby Jessica" drew feverish attention in 1993 when a child placed with adoptive parents was ordered by the Michigan Superior Court to be returned to her biological father, who had not been aware of her existence. The case created scrutiny of the rights of birth parents, increasingly birth fathers, and, some would argue, accelerated efforts by prospective adoptive parents to seek out intercountry adoptions (Collinson, 2007). Further, some would assert that fathers are stereotyped to be uncaring individuals who often advocate for terminating the pregnancy. Unfortunately, evidence is extremely limited, but the evidence we do have negates these perceptions.

In one of the first studies to examine the birth fathers' role and perceptions of relinquishment, researchers found that most fathers relinquished because of their own unpreparedness to be a father and that the decision was made in the best interests of the child. Still, some fathers reported feeling pressured to relinquish their children (Deykin, Patti, & Ryan, 1988). Interestingly, 67% ($n = 125$) had engaged in search activities, and this was correlated with thoughts of taking their children back. More recently, Clifton (2012) performed in-depth interviews with 20 birth fathers in England to ascertain themes from the experiences of relinquishment. The most prevalent themes were feelings of humiliation and defeat. The author formulated a theory by dividing the fathers' social and emotional styles as being either shame-prone (vindicators: low likelihood of a rich relationship with the child; or resigners: future role with the child poorly developed) or guilt-prone (affiliators: engaged in building a distant relationship with the child; Clifton, 2012). Research in this area is much needed to better understand fathers' experiences throughout the process of child relinquishment, and hence support efforts toward healing.

Effects of Relinquishment on Birth Mothers and Fathers

As previously discussed, we understand the least about the effects of placement on birth parents, especially long-term effects. Some evidence, however, is important to reference to enable APNs to provide informed care. In one study, Memarnia and colleagues (2015) performed an interpretive phenomenological analysis by conducting in-depth interviews with seven mothers who had relinquished children 2 to 9 years before the interviews. Four overall themes emerged: The first, "no one in my corner," conveyed feelings of no support before and after the child was placed. Anger toward professionals and the perception that placement could have been avoided were noted. Powerlessness was also a common emotion. The second theme, "disconnecting from emotion," is a complex phenomenon that simultaneously describes significant emotions while being disconnected from feelings. Further, mothers reported experiencing tremendous guilt and self-harming through substance abuse to numb the emotions. When emotions were acknowledged, it was only for short periods. The third theme, "renegotiating identity," described the struggle over whom they were and, as the authors stated, their "internal struggle to reconcile being a mother but not a parent"

(p. 308). Some mothers felt a need to improve their lives and in so doing, decrease the sense of shame and guilt. "The children are gone, but still here" was the fourth theme derived from the interviews. Birth mothers in the study had contact with their children, despite the children being placed in foster care or being adopted. Myriad emotions were evoked when visits occurred, from anxiety to guilt and anger directed toward themselves.

An organization, Concerned United Birthparents, provides information and support for those individuals who have relinquished their children (see Exhibit 3.4). They provide support through an online presence and advocacy for parents who have released their children into the care of others. APNs' awareness of potential maladaptive and complex reactions are helpful to avoid stereotyping birth parents who have had children removed due to maltreatment or who have voluntarily created an adoption plan. For uninformed providers, falling into the trap of judging birth parent behaviors needs to be tempered with a full understanding of context and interpersonal dynamics.

EXHIBIT 3.4

CONCERNED UNITED BIRTHPARENTS

Concerned United Birthparents, Inc. (CUB) (www.cubirthparents .org/index.php) is a nationwide organization, incorporated in 1976, that supports birth parents who have relinquished a child. Saving Our Sisters is a program sponsored by CUB that seeks to provide support for unnecessary adoptions. CUB's mission is articulated as follows:

Concerned United Birthparents, Inc., provides support for all family members separated by adoption; resources to help prevent unnecessary family separations; education about the life-long impact on all who are affected by adoption; and advocates for fair and ethical adoption laws, policies, and practices.

CASE STUDIES: BIRTH PARENTS

□ □ □ □

CASE STUDY 1: FRANK

Frank just turned 65 years old and is looking forward to finally being able to retire. His original position was a long distance, over-the-road trucker. However, 10 years ago, Frank transitioned from driver to in-house company foreman due to hypertension, which included some occasional dizzy spells. His hypertension is well controlled on lisinopril 40 mg once a day every morning. In addition, Frank has an 8-year history of type II diabetes, which is managed with metformin 1,000 mg with his evening meal. Two months ago, his HgbA1c was 6.9%. He uses a home glucometer for daily blood sugar readings.

He has two adult children by his second wife, who are independent and live out of state. Married for 10 years to his current wife, Frank is content with this third marriage. His wife has encouraged him to attend church services regularly with her, which has helped him make sense of his spirituality.

He is being seen today for increasing dizziness by his primary care provider, an adult-gerontology nurse practitioner (A-GNP), Carol. During her assessment, Carol notices Frank is diaphoretic and has a rapid heart rate (100 beats/minute), and fast, shallow breathing (26 breaths/minute). His blood pressure reading is 150/90, which is higher than his last previously recorded measurements of 118/67, 124/72, and 120/64. He relates his recurring dizzy spells have started to get a bit worse recently and happen when he is under a lot of pressure at work. Occasionally, he will feel dizzy before going to bed. Frank is usually a "cut up," making jokes when he is seen in the clinic by Carol. At his previous visit, Frank described how he and his wife were going to take a trip on their motorcycles across the Midwestern states, visiting landmarks. Today, however, Frank is quiet, and when Carol inquires about the trip planning, Frank states it has been postponed. When Carol meets Frank's eyes, he becomes defensive and blurts out he "doesn't want to talk about it."

Carol nods and offers the objective feedback regarding his presentation and how it differs from previous visits. "I sense that you're preoccupied with something."

Frank's shoulders slump, and he apologizes, and then relates how a daughter he had "given up for adoption" 40 years ago, contacted him 2 weeks ago. Frank shares when the baby girl was relinquished, the adoption was closed, and he had no idea what had happened to her. At the time, his first wife and he were not getting along, and the marriage and pregnancy were difficult owing to lack of resources. He was bouncing around between jobs on the road, and neither one had their own place to live. They both agreed the baby would be better off with an adoptive family. Shortly after the birth, he and the baby's mother split up. After the divorce, he lost contact with his first wife, and although he wondered what had become of his daughter, he had no desire to contact her, saying: "I didn't want to risk messing up her life."

His major concerns were that his current wife and his two adult children from his second marriage had no idea he had relinquished a child to adoption in the past and that the adopted daughter would see him as a failure. When this daughter did contact him, they agreed to meet for lunch the following week. Frank's daughter also told him that in her search for her birth parents, she discovered her birth mother had passed away, which made Frank feel even worse. Now Frank is feeling out of control with fear, guilt, remorse, and, yet, excitement—"I can't believe this is happening."

APN Next Steps

Carol listens to Frank and implements therapeutic communication techniques: listening, summarizing, reflecting, and nonverbally communicating acceptance (open body language, leaning forward). Carol understands how important it is for her to remain nonjudgmental and supportive. Frank has to make some important decisions: how and when to disclose to his family he had fathered a child who had been placed for adoption 40 years ago.

After a few minutes, Carol has the medical assistant recheck Frank's vital signs: his breathing is normal (16 breaths/minute), and his pulse is regular (90 beats/minute). She listens to his heart and notes a normal, regular rate and rhythm. All lung fields are clear to auscultation bilaterally. His blood pressure remains slightly elevated (136/80), which, compared with his previous measurements, is still high for him, but lower than his initial blood pressure reading of

150/90. When Frank is ready to leave, he begins smiling and tells Carol that he has enjoyed his "therapy session." Carol decides to hold off on changing his antihypertensive medication or ordering additional tests for now, but schedules a follow-up appointment to reevaluate Frank in 2 weeks.

Two weeks later, Frank arrives for his appointment with Carol and is more somber than usual. He relates his dizzy spells have decreased significantly. His vital signs are within normal limits: blood pressure is 120/74, pulse is normal (88 beats/minute), and respirations are normal (16 breaths/minute). He has been monitoring his blood glucose daily using his home glucometer, and his blood sugar readings have been at 70 to 120 mg/dL. He also describes the emotional reunion he had with his adopted daughter and how he truly understands he and his first wife "did the right thing by giving her up." Telling his current family has been very difficult. With varying degrees of understanding, particularly from his adult children, Frank is feeling a sense of relief. His two adult children feel betrayed because they have been denied knowing about a half sibling for all of these years. It is going to be a journey, he told Carol, but he is glad his family finally knows about his first child.

Carol knows Frank has some work to do with his family. His developmental stage of ego integrity versus despair has been impacted by the reunion with his adoptive daughter (Erikson, Erikson, & Kivnick, 1986). Frank's need to make sense of suddenly being a parent to a daughter he had relinquished for adoption 40 years ago and integrating this decision into his current life needs to be processed. By being an adoption-informed caregiver, Carol is able to treat the patient in a holistic manner. She compared Frank's previous presentations such as his blood pressure, pulse, and respiratory measurements, the recurrence of his dizzy spells, and his change in demeanor with his current signs and symptoms. Carol is able to discern the physical symptoms Frank was experiencing were directly related to his current state of emotional distress.

Applying this process in Frank's care resulted in the best outcome possible; no changes in Frank's medications or additional testing were necessary. Taking the time to thoroughly investigate the disconnect between Frank's previous provider visits and the changes Carol was seeing during this most recent visit, Carol is able to offer support during a crisis, providing a path to moving forward not only for the patient, but also for his family.

□ □ □ □

CASE STUDY 2: JASMINE

It is the beginning of the spring semester for Jasmine, a 15-year-old freshman in high school. The school has a high rate of school-subsidized lunches with a student body coming primarily from at-risk households. Jasmine has been complaining of nausea and receives permission to leave class to go to the health office. There, she learns from the school nurse, Mary, she is at the end of her first trimester of pregnancy. Jasmine has suspected that she may be pregnant because she had missed her "periods."

Mary is a member of the National Association of School Nurses (NASN) and realizes how vulnerable Jasmine is on many levels: physically, emotionally, psychologically, and developmentally. Mary, a family nurse practitioner (FNP), also realizes that Jasmine is at risk for dropping out of school (NASN, 2015), and she intends to provide Jasmine with a multifaceted support plan. After Mary and Jasmine discuss the news of the pregnancy, Jasmine concedes to telling her mother and father about the baby that night. She also discloses to Mary that the father "doesn't want anything to do with her, now that he knows she's pregnant." Mary sets up a time to meet with Jasmine and her parents at the school in 2 days.

Jasmine and her parents arrive; the parents present as both tired and angry. The mother barely looks at Jasmine and announces, "Well, if she thinks I'm raising this child, she has another thing coming. I'm still raising my own kids." The father is silent and looks downward, nodding. Jasmine is tearful and states, "I don't want an abortion." She then relates how two of her friends have had abortions and seem different, sadder after they had terminated the pregnancies. Then, in a deflated way, she adds, "I don't know what to do. Maybe I'll raise the baby myself."

APN Next Steps

Mary attended training in 2012 given by the Infant Adoption Awareness Training Program (Children's Bureau, 2015; see Exhibit 3.5), and

---

EXHIBIT 3.5

THE INFANT ADOPTION AWARENESS TRAINING PROGRAM (IAATP)

As directed by Public Law 103-310, the U.S. Congress authorized specific activities pertaining to Infant Adoption Awareness (amended Public Health Services Act; title XII, Subtitle A). The IAATP, a federal initiative and funded by the Children's Bureau of the U.S. Department of Health and Human Services, was designed to present a third option to unintended pregnancies: placement of a child for adoption by training designated staff in eligible health centers. Many professionals believed that the adoption option or "ad-option" was not being discussed with birth parents who were making this critical decision. Terminating the pregnancy or raising the child were often the only two alternatives considered. Since the IAATP was initiated, thousands of health care professionals have participated in the training.

Funding for the full IAATP ended in December 2013; however, the National Council for Adoption, through a grant from the Children's Bureau, has designed free training for health care and adoption professionals to be delivered through Internet-based modules available at: http://considerthepossibilities.org.

---

she presents best practices in communicating that placement of her infant is an option for Jasmine and her parents. Mary discusses all the options Jasmine and her parents are considering. She knows that Jasmine's mother did not want to have the responsibility for raising another child, and that the family's faith is prolife. Mary initiates the option of adoption: "Have you considered placing your child for adoption?"

Jasmine discloses that she has not really considered it, but cannot think about never seeing her baby after giving birth. Mary explains that there are many ways contact with adoptive parents and the child is handled. Although open adoption agreements and covenants may not be legally binding between the birth and adoptive parents,

Jasmine can select a family with whom she feels comfortable. She can request they sign a contract that would outline contact between Jasmine and the child. Mary also informs Jasmine that some contact with the birth parent is most frequently in the best interest of the child. Mary refers Jasmine to the crisis pregnancy center and to a counselor there for more discussions about the options she is facing. She also ensures that Jasmine has contact with birth mothers who had made an adoption decision, and those who had not, so that she could make an informed choice. Mary also verifies that in the state of residence, Jasmine, despite being a minor, has the right to place her child for adoption without parental consent.

Throughout the rest of the school year, Mary provides emotional support to Jasmine, who decides to make an adoption plan. Jasmine stops by and talks to Mary about some of the taunts from her peers who do not understand how she can "give her baby up." Mary listens and is careful not to communicate in a way that could later be viewed as coercive in favor of adoption. She knows that this decision needs to be made freely by Jasmine with input from her parents. She allows Jasmine to talk about her emotions, and how it makes her feel when the baby moves inside her. Mary shares how special that feeling is and emphasizes, "It takes a lot of courage to continue to go to school every day." Mary assesses Jasmine's social support structure, and discovers Jasmine has one friend and her maternal grandmother who are offering emotional support to her.

Three months later, Jasmine delivers a healthy baby, who, through an adoption agency, is placed with adoptive parents that she selected. They were present at the baby's birth with Jasmine and her mother.

At the beginning of her sophomore year, Jasmine stops by to see Mary. Although Jasmine's face brightens when she describes holding her baby immediately after delivery, she becomes less animated as she comments, "I just don't feel the same." She says she feels "so old," and yet she relates that she is convinced it was the best decision she could have made.

Mary understands the critical need for support and the grief process Jasmine is experiencing. Jasmine discloses, "At times, I just feel so angry and sad. I guess when you're poor and young, you really pay for your mistakes."

Mary encourages Jasmine to contact her adoption agency to determine whether they sponsor a postadoption support group for birth parents. She also discusses disenfranchised grief with Jasmine and how she needs to feel her emotions, be mindful of them, and continue to find meaning in the experiences over the past year. They talk about the birth father and how Jasmine had been able to make peace with him, including him on the adoption contract for the open adoption.

Mary makes it a priority to check on Jasmine weekly over the next several months. Jasmine is able to show Mary pictures of her child that the adoptive parents sent her. Seeing how well cared for the baby is, how the adoptive parents have honored the open adoption agreement, and Mary's support and acknowledgment of her grief enables Jasmine to move forward with her life.

□ □ □ □

CASE STUDY 3: THE MILLERS

Emily and Bart, a biracial couple, have been together for about 8 months, and each has two children by previous relationships. Barely able to cover their monthly expenses, Emily discovers she is pregnant. She is also midway through the surgical technician program at her local community college and hopes that upon graduation, she can finally make a livable wage. Bart has recently been laid off from his job at an American automobile factory and has been helping a friend do small remodeling jobs. They are 2 months behind in their apartment rent and face possible eviction, and have been fighting more frequently about money and what to do about the baby. Bart reasons that one more mouth to feed "won't make that much difference," but Emily is leaning toward terminating the pregnancy. One night after a particularly vicious argument that almost turned violent, with Bart slamming his fist against the wall, Emily orders Bart and his two children out of the apartment. She calls the local crisis pregnancy hotline in desperation, and tells them she is considering all her options, including abortion and making an adoption plan. The crisis center staff meet with her over the following weeks and refer her to a reputable adoption agency for more information.

Two months later, Emily decides to make an adoption plan. She and Bart have broken up, and she has informed him of her decision to place the baby with adoptive parents. He wants to meet to discuss the decision, and ultimately agrees this is the best option. With the help of the adoption agency case manager, Emily selects a family she believes will respect an open adoption plan.

Emily has been seen on a regular basis by her certified nurse-midwife, Jenny. Emily begins bringing the prospective adoptive mother, Alexis, to the appointments. Emily is at the clinic for her 37th week check. Jenny measures the fundal height, takes Emily's weight, and checks for signs of edema in her hands, face, and ankles. A urine sample is checked for any abnormalities that might indicate signs of preeclampsia. Jenny also takes a vaginal swab for group B strep. She listens to the baby's heartbeat, letting Emily and then Alexis, listen as well. All tests are normal or negative, and the baby and Emily are progressing well. Jenny also educates Emily on the signs of true contractions versus Braxton-Hicks.

APN Next Steps

As Jenny finishes the prenatal check, she notices Emily appears increasingly sad. She turns to Emily and asks, "The delivery is getting closer, and I know this is your third pregnancy. Each one is different. What are your questions and concerns?"

Emily quickly looks at Alexis, and Jenny inquires whether Emily would like Alexis to leave so that they can finish the check-up. Emily declines and then begins to cry. She discloses how fearful she is about being alone after the baby is born. She has grown attached to the baby, singing to it and talking to it. Alexis also begins to cry and states, "I feel so guilty taking this child from you."

Jenny assures both women that she understands how much courage these disclosures have taken, and that the feelings are real and need to be discussed. She asks about their plans after the baby is born and the arrangements that have been agreed upon. Alexis tells Jenny that an open adoption agreement has been drawn up that she and her husband intend to honor throughout the life of the child. Jenny encourages both women to continue to dialogue and share their feelings with one another. She knows that an open adoption arrangement, although in the best interest of the child, can be more complex for the parents. Careful not to persuade or dissuade Emily from any decision, Jenny emphasizes how important it is for the women to communicate openly and honestly during this time and the upcoming weeks.

She assesses Emily's social support network and the current dialogue with Bart, who has begun to refuse Emily's calls and does not respond to text messages. Jenny notes how vulnerable Emily is without proper emotional support and being a single parent to her two children. However, Emily was able to finish the semester at school and has only one more semester before graduation.

Two months later, Jenny sees Emily after a normal vaginal delivery. After deep reflection and consideration, Emily proceeds with placement. Today, she arrives with a flat affect. Before performing a postpartum check, Jenny assesses Emily's emotional well-being and the resources she has been able to access. Emily states she has been feeling very sad with the stress of explaining the adoption to her other children. She has not attended any support group meetings that the adoption agency has in place for birth mothers because she feels "so ashamed." Jenny probes further about these feelings and listens carefully as Emily explains that the adoption plan was really selfish on her part so that she could finish school. She laughs, describing how she got "so drunk" last night so she would not have to "feel anything for at least a little while."

During the visit, Jenny determines that Emily is at risk for significant depression/grief and is coping in unhealthy ways. She assesses her alcohol intake and uses the SBIRT guidance to facilitate this. Physically, Emily's postpartum check is normal. Jenny asks if she has visited the baby, a little girl, Sophia. Emily says she has not, adding, "I don't think I could take it." However, Alexis has invited her to see the baby, honoring the open adoption agreement. Jenny sits next to Emily, leaning forward and encouraging her to attend a support group meeting. Jenny discusses the grief process and the loss of being able to parent the baby, and acknowledges her pain.

Jenny also asks Emily to reflect on how she reached the decision to create an adoption plan, reviewing the steps Emily had taken. She points out that Emily had considered all of her children's needs; the ability to finish school would create security and stability for her children under her care. Emily had taken good care of herself during the pregnancy so that the baby would be born healthy. She ensured that the baby girl, Sophia, was going to know her and her birth father, Bart, if he wanted that. She had created a relationship with Alexis before Sophia's birth that had allowed Alexis to feel secure enough to invite Emily to visit Sophia. Jenny emphasizes how much Emily had done to protect her child and ensure the welfare of her children at home.

Emily is able to make eye contact and promises Jenny to look into the support group. Jenny encourages Emily to look into the postadoption counseling that the agency offers; she also gives Emily the website of online support groups if that is more comfortable for her. They discuss whether Emily might find an antidepressant helpful. Jenny makes a follow-up appointment with Emily to ensure her well-being and to continue to discuss whether an antidepressant would be beneficial.

□ □ □ □

CASE STUDY 4: CHELSEA

At 34 years of age, Chelsea has just learned of her promotion as manager of the oncology team, late phase development, at a global pharmaceutical company, and that she is 8 weeks pregnant. When she was in her early 20s, she had terminated a pregnancy and could not shake off the feeling of regret afterward. Despite being raised in the Roman Catholic faith, she does not attend church, or feel close to her faith. Yet she does not want to go through with another abortion.

As one of five siblings growing up, Chelsea watched her mother sacrifice her own education and career as she cared for the children in a traditional marriage. Ultimately, her parents divorced after 28 years together, leaving Chelsea even more disillusioned with marriage and family life. Chelsea has been in several relationships through the years, but she always broke things off when they became too serious. She reconciles this with the feeling that she has not met the person she is supposed to be with for the rest of her life. Her pregnancy is the result of a night with an acquaintance, someone at a pharmaceutical conference whom she knew previously when he worked at the same company where she is currently employed. She felt it was her duty to contact him, and when she did, she told him of her decision to place the child with a couple who desperately wants a child. He agreed and asked that she keep him posted on what would happen next—that he had heard of "open adoption" agreements, where the birth parents are allowed contact with the adoptive parents and the child.

Chelsea is a tall, thin person, and has successfully hidden her pregnancy into the last trimester. At that time, she arranges for family medical leave, citing an ill relative who needed her to help. The company is happy to provide 4 months of leave, given her stellar performance. Chelsea sees a certified nurse-midwife, Susan, for her prenatal care, whose practice is in a neighboring community.

APN Next Steps

Susan has guided Chelsea through her pregnancy; the patient is now in her third trimester, gaining an appropriate amount of weight, normal blood pressure, and no evidence of gestational diabetes or signs/symptoms of preeclampsia. The patient reports lots of activity from the baby and feels "like a cow" with all the weight gain. Susan's only concern is that Chelsea has a very limited support system: one old high school "best friend," who will be with her in the delivery room. During her week 36 visit, Chelsea discloses her plans to relinquish the child to a couple from out of state. She is a client of a reputable adoption attorney as she wanted the arrangement kept as confidential as possible. The father is willing to sign relinquishment papers upon birth, and they have entered into an open adoption contract with the prospective adoptive parents, which allows them face-to-face contact with the child.

Susan listens as Chelsea describes the arrangements in a matter-of-fact way and how she will return to work about 4 weeks after birth. Plans are made for her to deliver in the hospital in a city adjacent to where she resides. She does not allow the prospective parents in the labor and delivery room, but her friend is there to help her through her contractions and delivery. Chelsea gives birth to a healthy, 7.5 pound infant girl, and the process unfolds without any complications. She is given a private room at the hospital and, after she holds the baby immediately after delivery, Chelsea declines seeing her daughter again, stating: "She belongs to them now." She completes a medical history form for the adoptive family so that they have information about their daughter's health background. The hospital nurse offers Chelsea a follow-up call to check on her, but she declines.

Follow-Up

Chelsea sees Susan for her 6-week postpartum check and has a gynecological exam. Her milk has "dried up," and she feels great physically. Susan counsels her on PPD and birth control methods she might consider. Chelsea nods, and appears to understand.

Susan pauses, sensing something has not been said. Then Chelsea discloses that she drives 5 hours to see the baby weekly because she has that right given the open adoption agreement. Suddenly, she becomes agitated because during the last visit, the adoptive mother, Charley, had begun to cry, saying that she could not feel like Katherine's (the baby) "real mom" with Chelsea in the environment. She told Chelsea that she believed Chelsea was grieving and that Chelsea needed to seek a therapist to deal with her grief and loss, and learn to deal with the relinquishment. The adoptive mother emphasized that she would honor the open adoption contract, but was concerned for both of them.

Susan leans forward and sits facing Chelsea who is sitting up also. "Tell me what you're feeling right now."

"Oh, my gosh! So many things. I guess sadness, guilt . . . I'm wondering who I am. I've never felt this." She then begins to quietly sob with her head in her hands.

Susan understands that relinquishment of a child is one of the most difficult experiences for many birth parents, even when a birth mother, such as Chelsea, is sure it is the best decision for her and her child. But she also understands that Chelsea has had significant hormonal shifts and, as importantly, lacks a support system that would support her emotions and the experience. She is concerned about PPD, and understands that one of the major constructs in Cheryl Beck's Theory of Postpartum Depression is "loss of self" (Beck, 2002). Because Susan grasps the complexities of Chelsea's situation—physical, social, emotional, and psychological—she knows there is a need to refer Chelsea to a therapist who also is adoption informed to offer Chelsea the help she needs.

In that moment, however, Susan understands that she can offer comfort and support. "This must be overwhelming for you. Tell me about Katherine."

Chelsea looks up, "Oh, she's wonderful!" She looks down. "I know I made the right decision. I just never expected these feelings."

"Feelings. . ."

"Yeah, like sadness, happiness, peace, guilt, joy, acceptance, sadness, sadness, sadness. . ."

"So much to process." Susan waits and then asks, "What about the adoptive parents? What are they like?"

Chelsea swallows, but continues to wipe away tears. "They're great. They've been so patient with me. I just show up, you know? I tell myself not to go there, but I can't help myself. It's as much for me as for Katherine. There's no one I can really talk with, and Charley, the adoptive mom, is so kind to me."

Susan places her hand on Chelsea's arm. "You've been through a lot. And your body has been through a lot. You're healing inside and out. But we need others in our lives to help us sometimes. Would you be open to talking with a therapist, someone who can help you make sense of all this?"

Chelsea hesitates. "Do you know someone?"

Susan goes on to explain that she is aware of a very caring and competent therapist who has counseled many individuals whose lives have been touched by adoption. She urges Chelsea to make an appointment, and to "be gentle with yourself." The advanced practice nurse also describes "entrustment ceremonies," arranged between the birth and adoptive parents to signify the change in parentage (Child Welfare Information Gateway, 2013b). Susan prescribes an SSRI antidepressant for Chelsea, educating her that it will take 2 to 3 weeks for her to feel relief. She encourages Chelsea to call her if she needs additional information. A follow-up appointment is set for 4 weeks.

Susan knows that signs of PPD and grief may be intertwined. Chelsea's hypervigilance of Katherine may be both a sign of PPD and the grief process. When Susan sees Chelsea again, she will assess whether the antidepressant is helpful and whether Chelsea has entered into therapy.

□ □ □ □

APNs' Care of Birth Parents

These case studies are just a few of the possible narratives that are unique for birth parents. However, these case studies represent common issues that birth parents face who have released a child into the care of adoptive parents. Despite common issues, birth parents'

TABLE 3.2 *Birth Parents: What to Look for and What to Do*

Birth Parents

What to Look for (Assessment):

☐ In voluntary relinquishment, ensure that there is informed consent related to the decision to place the baby (e.g., no fees paid to the birth mother that would be construed as coercive).

☐ Verify state laws for minors who become pregnant, and consider adoption as a third choice for an unintended pregnancy.

☐ Monitor for signs of postpartum depression as well as grief (disenfranchised) and other mood disorders in birth parents.

☐ Assess social support for both birth mothers and fathers.

☐ Tease out physical complaints that may be related to psychosocial needs.

☐ Use SBIRT (Screening, Brief Intervention, Brief Therapy, and Referral to Treatment) guidelines to screen and intervene for substance use.

What to Do (Management):

☐ Consult organization's and state's reporting guidelines for reporting substance abuse and use in pregnant women.

☐ Provide psychosocial support and therapeutic communication during and after decisions to release the child for adoption.

☐ Advocate for birth parents' rights, and understand that relinquishment of a child is not an occurrence that ends when physical custody is released; rather, it is a lifelong process.

☐ Refer to adoption-informed mental health professionals when needed.

situations are heterogeneous and require the APN to individualize the approach, assessment, and plan of care. Priorities include the safety and well-being of the dyad and newly created families established through open adoptions. Safety issues may include substance use while the birth mother is pregnant, self-harm when depression is severe, and domestic violence. We discuss involuntary termination of parental rights further in Chapter 7. Table 3.2 provides guidance in areas that require APN assessment and management.

CHAPTER HIGHLIGHTS

☐ The number of unintended pregnancies ending in abortion has decreased, and births resulting from unintended pregnancies have increased; however, fewer infants are being released for adoption.

☐ Relinquishment of a child and the subsequent termination of parental rights may be voluntary or involuntary.

☐ Critics argue that termination of parental rights based on inadequate financial and social resources is an invalid reason to relinquish a child, and call this "unnecessary adoptions."

☐ In certain countries, such as China and India, female infants and children are often abandoned or released for adoption at higher rates than male infants and children. These practices are rooted in cultural practices and the value placed on sons.

☐ Safe Haven laws are designed to protect birth parents from criminal prosecution for abandonment; however, the infant must be left in a safe place designated by law.

☐ AWHONN and ACOG oppose laws that criminalize pregnant women for substance use disorders because evidence shows them to be ineffective deterrents to substance abuse. APNs should check state laws for mandatory reporting.

☐ Screening, Brief Intervention, Brief Therapy, and Referral to Treatment (SBIRT) appears to be an effective and efficient method in primary care in screening for and referral for further evaluation of unhealthy substance use.

☐ The Infant Adoption Awareness Training Program has been adapted by the National Council for Adoption, and this training for health care professionals is available online, free of cost.

☐ The continuum of contact between birth parents and adoptive parents extends from closed to open adoption. Open adoptions are the current norm and are considered to be in the best interest of the child. Legal enforcement of contact agreements varies by state.

☐ The effect of relinquishment of a child on birth fathers has been overlooked in both research and, in some cases, practice.

☐ Health care organizations have specific policies and procedures that are followed when termination of parental rights occurs in postpartum units. BUFA or "baby up for adoption" has been used to signify a baby who is being placed with adoptive parents.

☐ APNs and bedside nurses are influential during this fragile time and should avoid making judgments, swaying parties, or showing bias. Therapeutic communication, advocacy, and openness to grief reactions in birth parents are important interventions.

Questions for Reflection

Following are a few questions to reflect upon. You can use these to start a journal for yourself or in a classroom discussion with peers and the instructor.

1. How do race, class, and gender influence birth parents' decisions to relinquish a child?
2. What are your attitudes toward impaired birth mothers who endanger or permanently impact the health of their child? Where do the rights of the birth parents end and those of the child begin?
3. Have you ever been in a situation where it was difficult to remain neutral and still advocate for birth parents' rights?
4. What therapeutic communication techniques do you use when interacting with a birth parent who is experiencing disenfranchised grief?
5. What are your thoughts on open adoption contracts? Should they all be legally binding documents? What if the child's safety becomes a factor?
6. Which case study spoke to you the most? Why? What personal and professional feelings were evoked within you?

References

American Congress of Obstetricians and Gynecologists. (2011/2014, January). Substance abuse reporting and pregnancy: The role of the obstetrician and gynecologist (Committee Opinion, No. 473, 1–2). Retrieved from www.acog.org/Resources-And-Publications/Committee-Opinions /Committee-on-Health-Care-for-Underserved-Women/Substance-Abuse -Reporting-and-Pregnancy-The-Role-of-the-Obstetrician-Gynecologist

American Congress of Obstetricians and Gynecologists. (n.d.). Toolkit on state legislation: Pregnant women & prescription drug abuse, dependence and addiction. Retrieved from www.acog.org/-/media /Departments/Government-Relations-and-Outreach/NASToolkit.pdf

Association of Women's Health, Obstetric and Neonatal Nurses. (2015). AWHONN position statement: Criminalization of pregnant women with substance use disorders. *Journal of Obstetric, Gynecologic, and Neonatal Nursing, 44*(1), 155–157. doi:10.1111/1552-6909.12531

Beck, C. T. (2002). Postpartum depression: A metasynthesis. *Qualitative Health Research, 12*(4), 453–472.

Child Welfare Information Gateway. (2013a). *Regulation of private domestic adoption expenses.* Washington, DC: U.S. Department of Health and Human Services, Children's Bureau.

Child Welfare Information Gateway. (2013b). *Impact of adoption on birth parents.* Washington, DC: U.S. Department of Health and Human Services, Children's Bureau.

Child Welfare Information Gateway. (2013c). *Openness in adoption: Building relationships between adoptive and birth families.* Washington, DC: U.S. Department of Health and Human Services, Children's Bureau.

Child Welfare League of America. (1960). *Child Welfare League of America standards for services to unmarried parents.* New York, NY: Author.

Children's Bureau. (2015). *Infant adoption awareness training program.* Retrieved from www.acf.hhs.gov/programs/cb/resource/adoption -awareness-traning

Clifton, J. (2012). Birth fathers and their adopted children: Fighting, withdrawing, or connecting. *Adoption and Fostering, 36*(2), 43–56.

Collinson, A. (2007). The littlest immigrants: Cross border adoption in the Americas, policy and women's history. *Journal of Women's History, 19*(1), 132–141. doi:10.1353/jowh.2007.0007

Deykin, E. Y., Patti, P., & Ryan, J. (1988). Fathers of adopted children: A study of the impact of child surrender on birthfathers. *American Journal of Orthopsychiatry, 58*(2), 240–248. doi:10.1111/j.1939-0025.1988tb01585x

Erikson, E., Erikson, J., & Kivnick, H. (1986). *Vital involvement in old age.* New York, NY: Norton.

Finer, L. B., & Zolna, M. R. (2014). Shifts in unintended pregnancies in the United States, 2001–2008. *American Journal of Public Health, 104*(S1), S43–S48. doi:10.2105/AJPH.2013.301416

Foli, K. J. (2012). Nursing care of the adoption triad. *Perspectives in Psychiatric Care, 48*(4), 208–217. doi:10.1111/j.1744-6163.2012.00327.x

Guttmacher Institute. (2016, March). *State policies in brief: An overview of minors' consent law.* New York, NY: Author.

Manley, K. L. (2006, Winter). Birth parents: The forgotten members of the international adoption triad. *Capital University Law Review, 35*(2), 627–661.

Memarnia, N., Nolte, L., Norris, C., & Harborne, A. (2015). "It felt like it was night all the time": Listening to the experiences of birth mothers whose children have been taken into care or adopted. *Adoption and Fostering, 39*(4), 303–317. doi:10.1177/0308575915611516

National Association of School Nurses. (2015). Pregnant and parenting students: The role of the school nurse [Position statement]. Retrieved from http://www.nasn.org/Portals/0/positions/2015psparenting.pdf

Office of National Drug Control Policy & Substance Abuse and Mental Health Services Administration. (2012). *Screening, brief intervention, and referral to treatment (SBIRT)*. Retrieved from permanent.access.gpo.gov/gpo32077/sbirt_fact_sheet_ondcp-samhsa_7-25-111.pdf

Providers' Clinical Support System for Opioid Therapy. (n.d.). What we do. Retrieved from pcss-o.org

Roberts, L. R., & Montgomery, S. B. (2016). JCN: Online extra: India's distorted sex ratio: Dire consequences for girls. *Journal of Christian Nursing, 33*(1), E7–E15. doi:10.1097/CNJ.0000000000000244

Siegel, D. H. (2012). Growing up in open adoption: Young adults' perspectives. *Families in Society: The Journal of Contemporary Social Services, 93*(2), 133–140. doi:10.1606/1044-3894.4198

Siegel, D., H., & Smith, S. L. (2012). *Openness in adoption: From secrecy and stigma to knowledge and connections.* New York, NY: Evan B. Donaldson Adoption Institute.

Sisson, G. (2015). "Choosing life": Birth mothers on abortion and reproductive choice. *Women's Health Issues, 25*(4), 349–354. doi:10.1016/j.whi.2015.05.007

Wasserstrom, J. (1984). Resistance to the one-child family. *Modern China, 10*(3), 345–374.

Wolfgram, S. M. (2008). Openness in adoption: What we know so far—A critical review of the literature. *Social Work, 53*(2), 133–142.

4

Adoptive Parents

□ □ □ □

PURPOSE OF THE CHAPTER

In this chapter, the adoptive parent's role is described and discussed as the adoption process unfolds and the child enters into the family system. Often viewed as the member of the adoption triad with the least loss experienced, today's adoptive parent may have struggled with infertility and turned to adoption as a way to build their families. Still others already have children in the home (Jones, 2009) and pursue adoption as a way to build their families, regardless of their ability to procreate. As with other members of the triads, stereotypes abound about adoptive parents—from saints to sinners. Many parents describe being told, "You are a wonderful person to do this!" or, "I could never do what you're doing."

In contrast, the media is swift in pointing out heinous crimes of maltreatment rendered by adoptive parents. In instances of unregulated custody transfers, this coverage is well deserved. Unregulated custody transfers occur when adoptive parents hand over their children to strangers after advertising their children's availability on social media (this practice is discussed in depth later in this chapter). An investigative report published by Reuters on September 9, 2013, described these unconscionable transfers of internationally adopted children to other "parents," placing these children at great risk for harm. The adoption community and the world took notice, and the focus on postadoption support has become even more imperative.

What most adoptive parents are, however, are parents. They struggle in most respects with challenges as any parent would. But there are differences. In addition to the health status of adoptive children differing from children overall, there is a dynamic layer to the adoption journey that is threaded through the parent–child relationship. Parents approach this layer in different ways, sometimes contingent on what the child expresses—or does not express. There are also behaviors the child exhibits related to being an adopted person, which we discuss in the respective chapters on adopted children and kinship children (Chapters 5 and 8).

In this chapter, four narratives of adoptive parents are highlighted: a women in her late 30s who decides to breast feed her infant; a same-sex couple with a sibling group, one of whom is HIV+; a single mother who is struggling with depressive symptoms after her child is placed in her home; and a couple who is faced with a failed adoption. Each case describes the interactions parents have with their advanced practice nurses (APNs), followed by the identified issues and concerns that are amenable to nursing interventions.

Learning Objectives

At the completion of the chapter, the reader will be able to:

1. Articulate the common demographic patterns of adoptive parents, with an awareness of the heterogeneity of these parents
2. Describe challenges that are common to adoptive parents, including the stress of the adoption process, multiple uncertainties during the transition from pre- to postplacement, and integration of the child into the family unit
3. Identify signs and symptoms of depressive symptoms within the context of expectations and Foli's midrange theory of parental postadoption depression
4. Become skilled in therapeutic interactions with adoptive parents and the nursing interventions needed during the transition from pre- to postplacement
5. Explore ethical considerations of adoption as they relate to individuals who receive children

6. Establish an accurate vocabulary that describes placements that are interrupted, terminated, or fail

WHO ARE ADOPTIVE PARENTS?

Demographically, the 2 million adoptive parents, when compared to nonadoptive parents, have more education and higher incomes, are more likely to have been married, are older, and are typically White (Jones, 2009; Vandivere, Malm, & Radel, 2009). Sixty-nine percent of adopted children live with two married parents (Vandivere et al., 2009). But this profile should be tempered with an emphasis that many adoptive parents are not reflected by these demographics. Interestingly, adoptive parents reside in rural areas at a higher percentage than the general population (24% vs. 19%, respectively; Vandivere et al., 2009; U.S. Census Bureau, 2010). Anecdotal reports indicate that many adoptive families choose to live in such areas because of lower housing costs, more space, and in general, greater affordability (Wright, 2011).

Same-Sex Adoptive Parents

There are approximately 690,000 same-sex couples living in the United States (Gates, 2014). Of these couples, lesbian, gay, bisexual, and transgender (LGBT) individuals are a significant group of adoptive parents. Indeed, in the United States, approximately 22,000 children are being raised by 16,000 same-sex couples—couples who are four times more likely than different-sex couples to have adopted a child and six times more likely to be raising foster children. Compared to 3% of different-sex couples, 13% of same-sex dyads have an adopted child under the age 18 (Gates, 2013). This group of parents has been the subject of controversy with researchers examining the impact, if any, on their adopted and fostered children.

There is much to learn and select studies are highlighted here so that the APN may understand the scope of evidence collected thus far. The Donaldson Adoption Institute surveyed 1,616 adoptive gay and lesbian parents to determine their unique experiences and needs in a nationwide project called the Modern Adoptive

Families (MAF) Study (Brodinsky, 2015). A sub-set of these data were used by Brodinsky and Goldberg (2016a) to determine contact with birth parents headed by different- and same-sex parents. The authors found that for child welfare adoptions, same-sex parents had more contact and tended to have more positive relationships with birth families than heterosexual parents (Brodinsky & Goldberg, 2016a, 2016b).

Depressive and anxiety scores of gay and lesbian couples across the pre- to postplacement time period were examined in light of support and contextualized within the concept of stigmatized sexual orientation (Goldberg & Smith, 2011). Support from the workplace and family and relationship quality were related to lower depressive symptoms and anxiety at the time of the adoption. Lower internalized homophobia, higher neighborhood friendliness, and positive legal climates were related to lower depressive symptoms (Goldberg & Smith, 2011). Similarly, using the National Survey of Children's Health dataset, Bos, Knox, van Rijin-van Gelderen, and Gartrell (2016) found that for female same-sex households, although there were no differences in child outcomes (e.g., general heath, emotional difficulties, coping behavior, learning behavior) when compared with heterosexual households, same-sex couples reported higher parenting stress. The researchers were unable to determine the cause of this parenting stress and hypothesized that it may be related to the burden of sexual orientation stigma and having to justify parenting as same-sex couples (Bos et al., 2016). These hypotheses seem to be supported in a study of lesbian comothers conducted by Cherguit, Burns, Pettle, and Tasker (2013). Most mothers had positive experiences with maternity staff; however, structural issues still reflected heterosexism attitudes.

APNs need to be aware of sexual minority stigma, the hesitation of same-sex adoptive couples to share sexual orientation with others, and the potential for increased parenting stress. Legal and social climates affect same-sex couples and resources for these families are important. Resources for same-sex parents are available on the Internet as these couples build their families through adoption (see Exhibit 4.1).

EXHIBIT 4.1
RESOURCES FOR SAME-SEX PARENTS

Family Equality Council

"Family Equality Council connects, supports, and represents the three million parents who are lesbian, gay, bisexual, transgender and queer in this country and their six million children."

Source: www.familyequalitycouncil.org/about_us

COLAGE

"COLAGE unites people with lesbian, gay, bisexual, transgender, and/or queer parents into a network of peers and supports them as they nurture and empower each other to be skilled, self-confident, and just leaders in our collective communities."

Source: Reprinted by permission of COLAGE, www.colage.org.

PFLAG

"PFLAG is the nation's largest organization uniting people who are LGBTQ with parents, families, friends, and allies. With 200,000 members and supporters, and local affiliates in more than 350 communities across the U.S. and abroad, PFLAG is the largest grassroots-based organization of its kind. PFLAG is a nonprofit organization and is not affiliated with any religious or political institutions."

Source: www.pflag.org

Motivation to Adopt

The motivation to adopt is also very individualized. Some parents approach adoption as a way of building their family because of an inability to have children, such as when fertility treatments have been exhausted, or the parents may be sexual minority couples who choose to have children, or single individuals who long for children but are not partnered. Still other parents choose adoption with intention and a plan from the time they begin their courtship, perhaps as a result of having adoption or foster care as part of their family of origin or as a faith-based decision. Finally, some parents choose to adopt a child because they desire a specific gendered child and already have children in the home. They do not feel "that their family is complete yet."

Parents themselves report on the two major reasons why they adopt: to give a child a permanent home and to expand their families (Vandivere et al., 2009). Yet parental motivation to adopt also varies by type of adoption (see Figure 4.1). Parents who choose intercountry adoption report higher motivation to expand their families (92%), and provide a permanent home for the child (90%) than parents who choose foster care or private adoption. The experience of infertility is also higher for intercountry adoptive parents than for foster care and private domestic adoptive parents (Vandivere et al., 2009).

For same-sex couples, motivation to adopt includes the lack of being motivated by "biogenetic kinship" (Jennings, Mellish, Tasker, Lamb, & Golombok, 2014, p. 221). Adoption for both gay and lesbian couples encompasses feeling morally right about being able to provide a stable, autonomous, and legally protected home for the child,

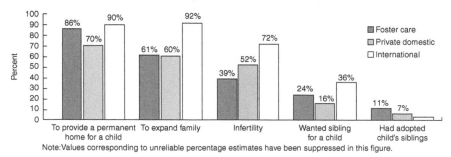

FIGURE 4.1   *Motivation to adopt by adoption type.*

Source: Vandivere et al. (2009).

as well as being free from involvement of other parties (Jennings et al., 2014). In sum, same-sex parents preferred adoption over other routes to parenting.

For adoptive parents, the primary motivator should not be to "save a child." Certainly there is a desire to provide the best possible future for a child, but this desire should be based in providing a home and building a family. To want to "save" a child assumes that there is a power gradient and an unspoken expectation of long-term gratitude from the child to the parents. To save something is usually a one-time event with the implication that you are saving the person from something or someone. In adoption, that something or someone is unclear, and if the adoptive parent is not thoughtful, there may be an undertone of cultural superiority. This position discounts the birth parents' decision to relinquish the child by creating judgments that one belief system is superior to another. When you adopt a child, it is a lifetime commitment to love a child as you would any child whom you are privileged to parent.

When a child is brought into a family unit, the couple needs to be in agreement with that decision. There is often a "dragger and dragee syndrome" when one parent is more enthused than the other and in turn, carries the majority of the responsibility for the child (James, 2009, p. 22). This lopsided approach to adoptive parenting can strain the relationship, potentially destabilizing the family. It is important—as with any major decision impacting the family—that both partners discuss and mutually agree upon if, how, and when a child is brought into the family. Unique stressors and risks to the marriage exist that stand in contrast to nonadoptive couples such as periods of infertility, lack of social support, and challenging behaviors of the child. There may also be buffers: higher socioeconomic status, being older and more educated, being married longer, and wanting to build a family through adoption. South, Foli, and Lim (2012) examined marital satisfaction in 251 adoptive mothers and found that socioeconomic status, partner support, enthusiasm of being a parent from the partner, and feeling rested predicted relationship satisfaction. Interestingly, infertility and the adoption process were not found to be related to relationship satisfaction. Thus, factors that are common to any parent appeared to be important to adoptive mothers in their relationships.

THE ADOPTION PROCESS

The bestselling series "What to Expect When Expecting," offers a fairly precise guide to the journey of pregnancy. However, given the various paths to adoption and that no national standards exist in vetting preadoptive parents, establishing a fixed timeline or description of what to expect in the adoption process is impossible. Yet, general steps are followed, regardless of the state in which the parent lives. First, there is a decision regarding the path to adoption: public domestic, private domestic, or intercountry (see Chapter 1). There is also an independent (private) adoption, in which an agreement between the adoptive and birth parent is reached without a third party such as a licensed adoption agency (however, attorneys may be used). Each type of adoption brings forward different dynamics and risks. For example, the amount of background information that is available or disclosed is often less with intercountry adoption. The age of the child may also vary, depending on the type of adoption, with private domestic adoptions usually placing infants, and public domestic adoptions placing older children.

Second, individuals who are interested in pursuing adoption need to determine who they will use to facilitate the adoption. For example, will they become foster parents in order to adopt through the child welfare system and the Department of Child Services (DCS), or will they employ the services of an adoption agency or private attorney (as in an independent adoption)? Depending on the type of adoption pursued and, thus, the professionals who will assist in the adoption, the costs will vary. Private adoptions that are facilitated through adoption attorneys are typically associated with the highest costs. Approximately 40% of all adoptive parents reported adoption expenses of $10,000 or more (Vandivere et al., 2009).

The least expensive (or no expenses) path to adoption is through the foster care system (public domestic). Select adoptions from foster care will have adoption assistance or subsidies available to parents after placement, especially in the cases of special-needs adoption. Adoption subsidies, at a median of $485 per month, help to provide for the child's basic needs as well as health care and therapies. These subsidies are often provided to foster parents (54%) and relatives (31%), who comprise the majority of parents who adopt from the public welfare system. Incomes of these parents are typically lower (less than $40,000) than those of the larger pool of adoptive parents. Positive associations between adoption rates and subsidies have been found (Evan B. Donaldson Adoption Institute, North American Council on Adoptable Children, & Adoption Support and Preservation, 2012).

One step that is universal is the home study process. While the exact information that is obtained differs between states, the home study is spearheaded by a licensed social worker or caseworker (Child Welfare Information Gateway, 2015). Interviews, health and financial statements, and criminal background checks are included in this study, with the primary objective to provide evidence of the individual's ability to parent a child. Critics argue that the process lacks the depth necessary to impart that adoption is a lifelong process that will impact the entire family. Current proposed reforms call for national guidance to standardize the home study process.

The APN may be asked to complete a physical examination and/or sign a health statement that attests to the individual's physical ability to care for a child. This is important information to complete the adoption dossier. An open discussion between the APN and the prospective parent should occur, with the age of the parent and the presence of chronic illnesses as considerations in planning to raise a child.

After the home study is complete, the prospective parent(s) wait for referral and/or placement of a child. In open domestic adoptions, preadoptive parents may accompany the birth parent during the pregnancy check-ups (see Chapters 1 and 3). For the APN, it is important to understand the dynamics of what open adoption means to the adoption triad and, ultimately, what it means to the child. Acceptance and understanding of the birth and prospective adoptive parents' relationship are critical as both parties are feeling vulnerable. Loss and hope are intertwined in the relationship, and the APN's personal feelings must be recognized and reconciled prior to these interactions. Often, sympathy for the birth parent may be present, a feeling that is difficult to process, and may transform into resentment toward the adoptive parent. A "winner" and "loser" in the adoption triad then becomes a cognitive model that may interfere with the therapeutic relationship. Conversely, a birth parent who is not following appropriate guidance for optimal health of the fetus may also elicit emotions.

Preadoption Training

When adopting a child from another country, the Hague Convention requires the prospective parent to undergo training in specific areas. As outlined in the Convention, these areas include the intercountry adoption process, medical issues in children adopted from abroad, issues surrounding attachment and institutionalization of children, and the child's cultural and ethnic history. Several proprietary companies have formed to provide the required training, and parents are able to complete the training online. The APN should be aware of additional questions the parents may have and should reinforce and supplement the materials the parents received through the Internet-based training.

Intercountry adoptions also require primary provider services, which are not to be confused with primary *health care* provider services. In the adoption context, primary providers are required via the Universal Accreditation Act (UAA) of 2012 (Bureau of Consular Affairs, U.S. State Department, 2016). The UAA presents federal standards for adoption primary provider services so that adoptions are conducted uniformly between nonparticipating (non-Convention) and participating Hague Convention countries, to uphold the tenets of the Hague Convention and to ensure ethical arrangements as a child is adopted from abroad.

For domestic adoptions, the requirements vary by state, with some training that includes first aid and cardiopulmonary resuscitation. This provides the APN direction for assessing how well prepared the parents are for the child: Do they understand their own expectations, the potential issues of attachment and bonding from both the child and parent perspectives, how to care for a child of that age? Unlike birth parents, adoptive parents may postpone preparation for a child, especially if they have experienced a failed adoption, when a planned placement does not occur. Individuals who have experienced a failed adoption sometimes make the decision to defer preparations until the child is physically in their homes. This places both the parents and the child in vulnerable positions, and the APN's assessment of preparedness—from bottles to bedding to education about development—will be important to support the transition of the family.

The Wait for Referral and Placement

The wait for placement of a child may be days, weeks, months, or even years. Influences such as the age of the child (infant vs. older child), changes in international document requirements, and failed adoptions may change events rapidly for the waiting parent. When a referral of a specific child has occurred, the child starts to become real to the parents. Several levels of contact are possible—from pictures and videos of children in foster care or orphanages from sending countries to face-to-face contact with a child in an orphanage in a developing country, to being a foster parent, to being in the delivery room when a child is born. Therefore, the amount and type of contact vary considerably. Parents should be aware that despite preadoption intense contact, the dynamics of the placement may change when the adoption is finalized. The child's temperament, health, and reaction to permanency may affect how smoothly the family transitions. For example, the child may "test" parents to see whether their family truly is "forever."

A failed adoption often has a devastating effect on the waiting parent. Several reasons may account for why a placement fails. Perhaps the birth parents changed their minds about the relinquishment, or the child passed away unexpectedly, or another event precluded a child from coming to parents who expected them. Parents who have experienced a failed placement have likened it to a miscarriage or death of a child.

Placement of the Child

The experiences of formal placement of the child are affected by the places and spaces of physical custody transfers. Transfers may occur in the hospital when the adoptive parents are allowed to bring the infant home, or in a foreign hotel room thousands of miles from their home, or months prior when foster parents decide to legally adopt a child under their care. Physical placement of the child may be different from legal finalization of the adoption. Countries have different approaches to finalizing the adoption; if legal finalization does not occur in the child's country, adoptive parents must finalize the adoption in their state. The Interstate Compact on the Placement of Children (ICPC) within the United States is important to explain. In brief, when a child is being adopted, both the sending state and the receiving state must give approval. This reciprocity also applies if the adoption is disrupted: the child must be returned to his or her original state.

There may be instances when the adoption is not completed or if it has been finalized, it is broken. The former, which occurs prior to finalization, is called "disruption" (Child Welfare Information Gateway, 2012). The physical placement has happened, but not the legal finalization. In the latter, physical and legal finalization have both been completed, but the adoption is broken; dissolution has occurred (Child Welfare Information Gateway, 2012). Both disruption and dissolution result in the child being entered into the foster care system or adopted by new parents. As with other adoption statistics, precise figures are elusive. Currently, disruptions are estimated to occur in 10% to 25% of families; dissolutions are even more difficult to estimate since birth records are often closed when the adoption is finalized. The accepted range of dissolved adoptions is between 1% and 5% (Child Welfare Information Gateway, 2012). A new term, postpermanency discontinuity, has been suggested to describe occurrences when individuals/children leave placement after adoption or guardianship has been terminated prior to becoming adults (Rolock, 2015). The term is not meant to carry a negative connotation, and serves to provide a broader description of placements a child may experience after a legal permanence has been established and then left. In a study of 21,629 children who had been adopted or placed in guardianship from foster care, 13% experienced postplacement discontinuity (Rolock, 2015). Examples of children who would fall under this category would include kinship children whose guardianship has changed, or a child placed into foster care after adoption for needed services (Rolock, 2015).

There are a multitude of reasons that contribute to disruption, dissolution, and postpermanency discontinuity and include child, parent, family, and agency factors. APNs need to understand the heterogeneity of adoptive families, and provide patient-centered care when parents are considering disruption and dissolution. Safety and the well-being of the child and family should guide such a course.

Postplacement of the Child and Postadoption Services

The transition to integrating the child into the family includes not only the parents, but siblings and extended family members. Parents may be faced with expectations that have been met or exceeded, or ones that were unrealistic or unfulfilled. A transition occurs as the new family member is integrated into the social unit. Only recently has attention been given to families' ongoing challenges during the vulnerable postplacement period when almost 20% of families engage in family counseling and 57% of adolescents who were adopted from foster care receive mental health services (Smith, 2014; Vandivere et al., 2009). Many adopted children face adversities early in life, thus adoptive families often encounter subsequent challenges that highlight the national lack of postadoption services (Smith, 2010, 2013). A recent and comprehensive report conducted a state-by-state examination of publicly funded postadoption services, including uniformity of services within the states (Smith, 2014). The report found that at least 13 states have no postadoption services, with disparities in services provided to rural areas across the states (Smith, 2014). Postadoption support includes primary health care and adoption informed providers.

Trauma-Informed Parenting

Children who are adopted and under the care of adoptive and kinship parents have often experienced at least one type of trauma. In multiple areas of specialty, APNs can support and educate parents in understanding the dynamics of these traumatic experiences. Developmental stages, the chronicity of the trauma, family systems, and generational factors need to be taken into consideration as the trauma is discussed. Specialized information for traumatized children *and their caregivers* is available. Established in 2000, the National Child Traumatic Stress Network (NCTSN) is funded by the Center for Mental Health Services (CMHS), Substance Abuse and Mental Health Services Administration (SAMHSA), and U.S. Department of Health and Human Services, and is jointly coordinated by the University of California, Los Angeles and Duke University. Its mission is to "raise the standard of care and improve access to services for traumatized children, their families, and communities throughout the United States" (NCTSN, 2015). Several excellent resources are available to families, professionals, and health care providers, including APNs (see Exhibit 4.2). We discuss additional resources in Chapter 6.

EXHIBIT 4.2

NATIONAL CHILD TRAUMATIC STRESS NETWORK (NCTSN): RESOURCES FOR APNS

Broader than just helping with trauma associated with adoption and kinship families, the NCTSN provides many resources for APNs:

☐ *Types of traumatic stress (from community violence to traumatic grief)*

☐ *Products available via the NCTSN, which include print-ready brochures and educational materials related to childhood trauma*

☐ *The NCTSN Learning Center for Child and Adolescent Trauma, including training videos, blogs, podcasts, continuing education, and toolkits*

☐ *The NCTSN Empirically Supported Treatments and Promising Practices, factsheets that include the name of the treatment, target population, modality (individual/family), and training guidelines*

☐ *Medical trauma, with "Pediatric Medical Traumatic Stress Toolkit for Health Care Providers," "Medical Events and Traumatic Stress in Children and Families," and a NCTSN reading list of papers on medical traumatic stress*

TRANSITION OF ADOPTIVE PARENTS

The transition from childless individual or a parent with existing children in the home to an adoptive parent can be extraordinary. While the addition of any child in the home carries with it a transition, adoptive parents experience a unique journey, sometimes because of what they have experienced (infertility, failed adoptions, and long wait times for a referral) and sometimes because of the child's presence (unknown special needs, temperament, and interaction with siblings).

In a qualitative study, McKay and Ross (2009) analyzed in-depth interviews of adoptive parents (8 females and 1 male) to describe the transition to adoptive parenthood. They found that overall, parents

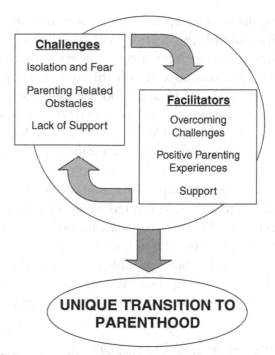

FIGURE 4.2   *Unique transition to adoptive parenthood: Conceptual framework.*
Source: McKay and Ross (2009).

experienced both challenges and facilitators, which were unique to adoption and to the parent (see Figure 4.2). For example, the parents understood that they were raising a child born to another person and felt acute responsibility to be perfect. Fear of losing the child was a theme identified as several of the parents had experienced a failed adoption. Infertility was also reported to affect the transition as couples had waited so long to have a child; being an older parent left them feeling without a peer group. Difficulty in expressing challenges to family and friends impeded receiving needed support. Facilitators were also cited, and as with the challenges, were unique to adoption: finally achieving their goal of becoming parents, seeing their child grow and cross developmental milestones, and seeking support, often from other adoptive parents (McKay & Ross, 2009).

    Fontenot (2007) integrated the findings from six studies that spanned pre- to postplacement of adoptive mothers. This integrative review pulled literature from 1990 through 2006, and findings parallel the facilitators and challenges identified by McKay and Ross (2009). For example *preadoptive* mothers reported "uncertainty, rejection, competition, isolation, judgment, apprehension, helplessness, risk taking, and fear, as well as fulfillment, hope, joy and love" (p. 180). In the *postadoption* time period, mothers expressed: "love, joy, happiness, and relief . . ., but uncertainty, sadness, isolation, unpreparedness, judgment, and fear" (p. 180). In a systematic literature review conducted by McKay, Ross, and Goldberg (2010), researchers revealed that only 11 studies had discussed mental health, physical health, and partner relationship satisfaction of adoptive parents. Due to the scant literature available, limited inferences were drawn from the studies reviewed. Tentative conclusions were that depression in the postadoption time period is relatively common; however, it is not as prevalent as in the birth parent population (McKay, Ross, & Goldberg, 2010). We will discuss the literature related to parental postadoption depression more fully in the following.

Adoption Disclosure and Discussion

With open adoption arrangements being more common, adoptive parents' disclosure about the child being adopted becomes non sequitur. Regardless, the adoption community agrees that the child deserves to know they were adopted. However, evidence indicates that the discussions surrounding the placement of the child creates unease for some adoptive parents (Wydra, O'Brien, & Merson, 2012). Adopted persons were dissatisfied with the disclosures when their parents were uncomfortable discussing their adoption narratives with them. Using books may be a strategy to open conversations with the child and ongoing discussions about being an adopted person and an adoptive family extend throughout the life of the child.

MATCHING

How are parents and children matched? Professionals in the adoption community have commented on what makes a strong match between a child and (adoptive) parent, and we have seen historical shifts in what matching entails. Today, there is growing consensus on what those elements should include. Historical matching of child-to-parent

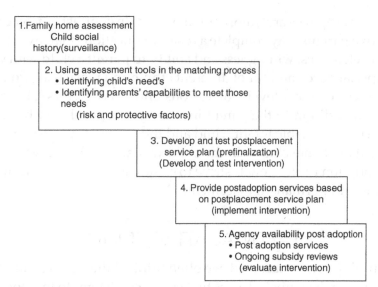

FIGURE 4.3   *Adaptation of public health model of prevention to adoption.*
Source: Hanna and McRoy (2011).

has been subjective and based on physical attributes. Today, matching has become more thoughtful with myriad assessment tools to support an optimal fit of parent and child. From conversations with adoption professionals, one consensus is that there is not enough attention paid to this critical step in the adoption process. The transition in adoptive practices from the "Baby Scoop Era" to enhancing permanency in placing a child was summarized by Hanna and McRoy (2011): "The shift in focus from finding a child for a family to finding a family for a child has meant a shift and an expansion of the matching process in adoption" (p. 62). The authors also described an overlay of the public health model of prevention: moving from child-to-parent/family matching to an assessment of stressors, and planning for services so that those stressors can be addressed (see Figure 4.3). Testing of this paradigm is needed. If such a model provided evidence of success, this may have significant implications for reducing disruptions, dissolutions, and displacements.

Elements of matching are also dependent upon the type of adoption pursued. In Chapter 3, we discussed how, in the cases of domestic private adoptions, social media has opened up new channels for birth parents to use as they select prospective adoptive parents by viewing webpages and information posted. In contrast, intercountry adoptive parents may complete a roster of questions that inventories their preferences, willingness and ability to parent a child with various special needs and/or of different ethnic and racial backgrounds, and assess comfort levels for various child risk factors. However, often, in addition to the parent inventory, a referral may be based on the next available infant/child and the parent's "place in line for the next available child." In the child welfare system, caseworkers and adoption professionals strive to ensure a match that will ensure a stable and permanent placement.

PARENTAL ATTACHMENT

When adoption is discussed, we often think of the child establishing a bond with the parents. Issues that create challenges to this bonding have been widely described in adoption research. However, in this section, the *parent-to-child attachment* is discussed, and as discussed here, is separated from child-to-parent bonding and attachment. Caseworkers typically assume an instant attachment from parent to child. However, this attachment may take time to develop (Foli & Thompson, 2004). Mother-to-child bonding was found to be an explanatory variable of depressive symptoms in 300 mothers who had adopted a child in the past 24 months. A significant relationship was found between lower bonding scores and higher depressive screening scores (Foli, South, & Lim, 2012a). Some parents have described a "fake it until you make it" strategy to give them time to establish a bond. Research into the relationship between parental attachment and disruption/dissolution is needed to craft nursing interventions to optimize permanency and to protect members of the family unit.

Private Rehoming

As mentioned earlier, in September 2013, Reuters news service published an explosive story on "private re-homing of children," especially those who had been adopted from other countries (Twohey, 2013). When a child is "rehomed," or experiences an unregulated custody transfer, adoptive parents transfer custody of the child to others, often strangers without government oversight. Such high-risk practices leave the child vulnerable to abuse and trafficking. Recently the Government Accountability Office (GAO) issued a report to address this horrific practice and, while the extent of the problem is unknown, identified precursors were difficulty accessing or financing postadoption support (GAO, 2015). Adoptive parents present several rationales for why they either post on Internet sites for "new parents" or use a middleman to do so: lack of resources to support parenting the child; extremely disruptive, sometimes violent behaviors exhibited by the child; and undisclosed special needs of the child that overwhelm the parents. Regardless, such practices are insupportable and place the child in grave danger.

When the parents present themselves to the APN, as either recipients of care or for their child's care, the APN should assess how the placement is proceeding. Warning signs of attachment difficulties from either the parents or the child should be pursued: poor eye contact, lack of interactions, angry or flat descriptions of child behaviors, verbalizations of the lack of needed services, unknown special needs of the child that have overwhelmed the family, suspected parent or child substance use, and financial strains due to the child's needs. While this not an exhaustive list, the APN should be aware that placement signifies a time of change and integration and may last months after formal adoption has occurred.

PARENTAL POSTADOPTION DEPRESSION (PAD)

In 1995, June Bond, an adoption professional and mother, explored her observations about a pattern of adoptive parents' behaviors that seemed to change after the child was placed in the home (Bond, 1995). She called it postadoption depression syndrome (PADS) and described the behaviors she saw in parents who had set themselves up to be super-parents and encountered other stresses related to parenting and adoption. This article was the first to give the depressive symptoms experienced by adoptive parents a name. In addition to scientists from other disciplines, I have attempted to understand depressive symptoms in adoptive parents. My book, *The Post-Adoption Blues: Overcoming the Unforeseen Challenges of Adoption* (coauthor John R. Thompson, MD, 2004), built on the notion that some adoptive parents struggle with depressive symptoms after the child comes home. Based on interviews with adoption professionals, parents and an expert in postpartum depression

(Dr. Cheryl Beck), a common and resounding theme that emerged was parental expectations. These expectations or beliefs in the future were expressed in several dimensions: expectations of themselves as parents, of their child, of family and friends, and of others (see Exhibit 4.3). My collaborators and I have carried Bond's work forward over the past 10 years and have conducted several studies that test whether parental expectations are indeed a correlation to depression.

EXHIBIT 4.3

PARENTAL EXPECTATIONS

Expectations of Self as Parent

Expectations of the adoption process
☐ *"I will have control over this process."*
☐ *"I have resolved all of my emotional pre-adoption issues."*
☐ *"The adoption process is complete once my child is placed."*

Parenting abilities
☐ *"We have to be the 'World's Best Parents'."*
☐ *"I will feel legitimacy as a parent."*
☐ *"I will feel like a real parent."*
☐ *"I will be able to keep every promise I have ever made to my child and her birthparents."*

Attachment to the child
☐ *"I will immediately feel that this is my child."*
☐ *"I will like this child."*
☐ *"If I maintain some emotional distance, I won't get hurt."*
☐ *"I will handle the changes in lifestyle that parenting brings."*

Expectations of the Child

The child's well-being
☐ *"My child will be okay."*
☐ *"My child's needs will be disclosed."*

(continued)

EXHIBIT 4.3 *(continued)*

The emotional needs of your child

☐ *"My child will like me, attach to me, and learn to love me."*

☐ *"My child will be as happy as I am."*

☐ *"My child's needs will be the same as those of other children."*

☐ *"My child's story is the same as our family's story."*

Making your child part of the family

☐ *"My child will be a good match for this family."*

☐ *"My child will behave in a consistent manner."*

☐ *"My child will respond to my parenting style."*

☐ *"My child will be integrated into our family."*

Expectations of Others

Expectations of family and friends

☐ *"Our child will be welcomed into the family."*

☐ *"I'll receive support in the same manner as I would with a birth child."*

☐ *"My family and friends will understand that our motivation and need to parent is the same as others' motivation and need to parent."*

Expectations of birthparents

☐ *"I will understand the birthmother's decision and circumstances."*

Expectations of society

☐ *"Society will respect the intimacy of my family,"*

☐ *"My community will offer a peer group for my child and me."*

☐ *"Society will support my decision to become an adoptive parent."*

☐ *"Society will include my family and me as equal members."*

☐ *"Professionals will treat adoptive families just like other families in society."*

Expectations of adoption professionals

☐ *"They will prepare me for the challenges I might face."*

☐ *"They will help me cope with any challenge I face."*

(continued)

EXHIBIT 4.3 *(continued)*

☐ *"They are there to get me a child."*

☐ *"They are there to give me a license to parent."*

☐ *"They will understand adoption and be competent in assisting me with the process."*

Adapted from Foli and Thompson (2004).

Foli's Midrange Theory of Parental Postadoption Depression

Since our book, *The Post-Adoption Blues*, was published in 2004, I have extended this construct of expectations and forwarded a midrange theory, which I have tested, refined, and supported through multiple empirical studies. My theory posits that because of the rigor and invasive nature of the home study process, as well as other factors that are unique to individuals who adopt (e.g., infertility, adopting an older child, history of child maltreatment, unknown medical/special needs of the child), adoptive parents may create expectations in dimensions (of themselves as parents, of the child, and of others) that may be unrealistic and later, unfulfilled. This disconnect or dissonance between expectations and reality may result in parents experiencing depressive symptoms (Foli, 2010).

I am often asked how PAD and postpartum depression (PPD) compare; my conclusion is that there are similarities and differences. First, the prevalence of new mothers who experience PPD is estimated to be between 10% and 15% (Gavin et al., 2005; O'Hara & Swain, 1996; Vesga-Lopez et al., 2008). For birth fathers, the prevalence of paternal PPD is estimated to be 10.4% (Paulson & Bazemore, 2010). In comparison, the rate of PAD in mothers ranges from 8% to 32%, with mothers surveyed in contexts of intercountry and domestic adoptions (Dean, Dean, White, & Liu, 1995; Fields, Meuchel, Jaffe, Jha, & Payne, 2010; Foli, South, & Lim, 2012a; Gair, 1999; Mott, Schiller, Richards, O'Hara, & Stuart, 2011; Senecky et al., 2009).

My team and I have found rates from 18% to 26% (mothers) and 11% to 24% (fathers) (Foli et al., 2012a; Foli, South, Lim, & Hebdon, 2012b).

Risk Factors and PAD

Cheryl Tatano Beck, DNSc, CNM, FAAN, who has written the foreword to this guide, has also advanced our understanding of PPD with her midrange theory and multiple research studies (e.g., Beck, 1996a; 1996b; 2002a; Kennedy, Beck, & Driscoll, 2002). Dr. Beck and colleagues also developed the Postpartum Depression Inventory-Revised (PPDI-R) to assess the risk of birth mothers developing PPD (Beck, 1998; 2002b; Beck, Records, & Rice, 2006). We used the PPDI-R with minor adaptations (i.e., changing "infant" to "infant/child") to determine whether the risk factors for developing depressive symptoms for birth parents were applicable to adoptive parents. After assessing 127 adoptive parents, we found four groups of parents who followed trajectories of risk before placement to 5 to 6 months after placement. One group (5% of the parents) had significant risk factors pre- and postplacement. However, there were additional risk factors not included in the PPDI-R that varied among parent groups, such as expectations of themselves as parents, of the child, and of family and friends; social support; ill temper; social anxiety; panic; traumatic intrusions; feeling rested; and differences in intimate partner relationships that require further investigations (Foli, South, Lim, & Hebdon, 2016a).

Longitudinal Course of PAD

To answer the questions of rate and course of PAD, we conducted a study of 129 primarily heterosexual parents and found five classes of depressive symptom trajectories of parents across time, from pre- to postplacement (Foli, South, Lim, & Jarnecke, 2016b). The good news is that most parents (71%) experienced only low levels of depressive symptoms, below the screening threshold of the Center for Epidemiological Studies-Depression (CES-D; Radloff, 1977). However, two classes were above the threshold at placement and three classes were above the threshold at 5 to 6 months postplacement (Foli et al., 2016b; see Figure 4.4). Implications for the APN include an awareness that

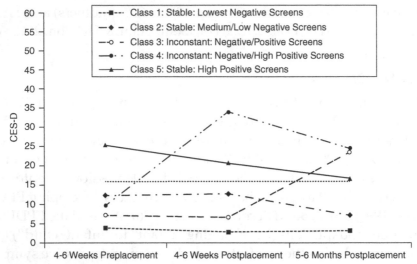

FIGURE 4.4   *Trajectories of depressive symptoms across time.*
Source: Foli et al. (2016b).

select individuals may enter the adoption process with depressive symptoms or may screen positive for depression after placement.

To be clear, far less is understood about the depression that some adoptive parents experience when compared with PPD. In the adoption community, there are varying levels of acceptance of PAD, with both skeptics and those that are convinced PAD does occur. Regardless, the evidence indicating negative outcomes for children who are cared for by parents—birth and adoptive—who experience depressive symptoms is compelling (Pemberton et al., 2010; Tully, Iacono, & McGue, 2008). When I am interviewed by journalists about PAD, I emphasize that when we address depression in parents, we are supporting the entire family. The common metaphor of when an airplane is losing altitude and oxygen is needed, placing the mask on the parent first so that the child can be helped, applies to parental postadoption depression as well. As with depression in the general population, social support is critical. Family and friends' support may not be as overt as when a family welcomes a birth child into the home. Transracial adoptions may pose challenges in relationships with extended family members. One adoptive mother shared how her grandfather could not accept her child from Asia because he was influenced by his service in the military.

Rykkje (2007) focused on the needs of transracial families and how "external categorizations" from strangers who commented on the differences in appearance between parent and child, were unexpected and annoying (p. 509). We found that mothers who adopted transracially did not differ in overall depressive symptoms from mothers who had not adopted transracially, yet they were less likely to perceive society had accepted them as a family (Foli et al., 2012a). We will discuss transracial adoptions again in Chapter 5.

Often the stigma and shame accompanying PAD is significant. Parents have reported "feeling like a monster" when bonding with the child is not instantaneous or they feel overwhelmed with the child's behaviors or special needs. They are hesitant to seek support given this is what "they wanted." APNs are in a key position to ensure that an open dialogue and nonjudgmental communication occurs when they sense a parent is struggling.

CASE STUDIES: ADOPTIVE PARENTS

□ □ □ □

CASE STUDY 1: JIM AND REGINA

The Stapletons decided to start a family 5 years ago. Both Jim, a 36-year-old financial advisor, and Regina, a 32-year-old middle school English teacher, came from large families and wanted to build one with each other. Three years passed without being able to conceive a baby and Regina experienced increasingly painful menstrual cycles. Fertility specialists confirmed Regina's diagnosis of "endometriosis-associated infertility," and the couple decided to pursue private domestic adoption as a way to build their family. After looking at various programs, they select an adoption agency to assist them in developing a webpage and have requested placement of an infant.

After 10 months, a 19-year-old African American birth mother, Makala, living a few hundred miles from them, selects them as potential adoptive parents. The birth father agrees with the adoption plan and remains Makala's partner. She insists upon an open adoption agreement, which the Stapletons' attorney assists in drafting. In their state of residence, the adoption agreement is not legally enforceable;

however, both couples firmly believe that the agreement should be honored. In the adoption contract, Makala has asked for "future contact, communication, and visitation." Jim and Regina send approved financial support for medical and living expenses while forging a relationship with Makala through Internet videoconferencing and occasional visits.

Regina goes to her primary care provider for her health statement; while there, she discloses that she would like to breast feed the infant, and she is referred to the certified nurse-midwife, Amy, an associate in the office.

APN Next Steps

Amy, a certified nurse-midwife, sees Regina for her first visit approximately 2 months prior to the couple's anticipated travel date to pick up their infant son. Regina confides how important breastfeeding their son is to her. Perhaps she feels this way, she admits, because of her infertility issues. She has never had a child and knows this might increase the challenges of inducing lactation and breastfeeding. But she is determined to try her best.

Amy listens carefully to Regina, understanding that support and education will be critical to successful breastfeeding. She assures Regina that the Association of Women's Health, Obstetric and Neonatal Nurses (AWHONN), National Association of Pediatric Nurse and Nurse Practitioners (NAPNAP) special interest group on breastfeeding, the American Academy of Pediatrics (AAP, 2005) and the American Academy of Family Physicians (AAFP, 2016) policy statements support adoptive mothers breastfeeding their children.[1] She also refers Regina to the La Leche League (La Leche League International, 2008–2016) for additional information and tips on breastfeeding. Amy discusses the use of galactagogues, both pharmaceutical and herbal, as well as a supplemental feeding device that loops around the mother's neck and provides additional nutrition to the infant as the infant sucks on the breast, thereby feeding and stimulating additional milk production. The device delivers supplemental formula that Regina can prepare and mix with her own milk, if there is enough produced.

---

[1] See specific policy statements for contraindications for women and breastfeeding.

Amy encourages Regina to begin using a breast pump eight times per day to induce lactation, but again advises that she may need to complement with other nutrition for the child through the supplemental feeding device. Amy also explains the supply of milk during induced lactation may not be an indicator of how much milk will be produced once lactation is achieved. The supplemental device has a small tube attached to it that allows the baby to simultaneously suck from both the nipple and the tube. In this way, the breast is stimulated to produce milk and the baby is ensured adequate nutrition.

Amy also enforces the emotional and psychological benefits of lactation will often be as important, if not more so, than the nutritional value of human breast milk. Understanding the bonding process for babies who are adopted, Amy knows Regina will be able to interact with her baby in a way that nonbreastfeeding mothers may not be able to. However, she strongly emphasizes that if the baby rejects the breast, it should not be construed as a rejection of her. The skin-to-skin contact, stimulation, and bonding between Regina and the baby are valuable, with or without the actual breastfeeding. Amy refers her to a lactation consultant in the community for further instructions and preparations.

Follow-Up

Four months later, Regina visits Amy for a follow-up visit and reports that her efforts with breastfeeding have been fairly successful between her own milk production and supplemental formula. Her baby, John, is now 6 months old, just starting on cereal and continuing to nurse on demand. Regina will be returning to teach school in the fall with plans to pump and freeze her milk when she cannot nurse John. Amy assesses for additional transition issues, such as parent-to-child and child-to-parent bonding, marital satisfaction, the "baby blues," and available support. Regina describes the emotional time spent with Makala and her partner and how the open adoption is working. There have been a few "bumps," but overall, they know this is in the best interest of John.

Glad the process is over, Regina is very grateful to the birth parents for giving life to John. She admits after being married without children, she and Jim experienced a transition. But, she adds, "It is all good!" and smiles. Her family has been less supportive than the couple's friends and coworkers, who have brought casseroles and planned a surprise baby shower for Regina. And she adds, "It was kind of hard at first to see John as ours."

Amy nods, "Being able to express these emotions is so important. It sounds as if you're making a solid transition with your new baby." She observes how Regina, when referring to John, speaks in a positive, animated way and is convinced the new mother is progressing well during this transitional period. They discuss Regina's plans to breastfeed until John is about 12 months before the visit concludes.

□ □ □ □

CASE STUDY 2: BILL AND EDDIE

Bill and Eddie fell in love 5 years ago when they met at their advertising firm in a state in the northwestern United States. In June 2015, after the Supreme Court struck down all states' bans on same-sex marriage, they were legally wed. Now, they are ready to take the next step in their lives and become parents. After discussions, they decided they want to become foster parents and adopt through the child welfare system. They intend to be matched with a child who is HIV positive. Eddie had a tough childhood and wants to make a difference in an older child adoption. The couple decides Eddie will stay home with the child, given that there will be health care appointments and other responsibilities. Both men go through the preadoptive training, including therapeutic foster parent training and background checks; provide references; have their medical forms signed; and complete the paperwork to foster. They meet with the caseworker who finishes several assessments with a child she has in mind for Bill and Eddie. The little girl, Cassie, who is 6 years old, is actually part of a sibling group; she has one younger sibling who is HIV negative (a girl, 4 years). The case worker discloses that the children have a history of maltreatment, but given their ages, the documentation is vague. They have been with their current foster family for 1 year and are fairly stable physically and emotionally.

The two children are placed with Bill and Eddie after health education is given regarding HIV and methods to protect members of the family from transmission of the virus. The education also covers ways to avoid exposure of opportunistic infections to Cassie. The children have been living with the couple for approximately 2 months when Eddie becomes ill with difficulty breathing and fatigue. He decides to go to his primary care provider, Kathleen, an adult-gerontology primary care nurse practitioner.

APN Next Steps

Kathleen is examining Eddie today for an upper respiratory tract infection. He presents with a low grade temperature, significant congestion in his sinus cavities with clear drainage, pharyngitis, and complaints of general malaise. He takes multiple vitamins and herbal supplements and works out three times per week.

After examining Eddie and deciding that the infection is viral, Kathleen advises on symptom relief: rest, fluid intake, over-the-counter decongestants, and nonsteroidal anti-inflammatory drugs (NSAIDs).

Eddie remains seated on the table. "Can you test me to see if I'm HIV positive?"

Kathleen is aware that he is the father to an HIV-positive child. "Tell me more about your concern."

"Cassie had a nose bleed, and I think I may have gotten some blood on my hand. I wasn't wearing gloves." He looks down.

"Yes, I can order that." Kathleen pauses and tries to meet Eddie's eyes. She pauses.

"It is tough, you know? I love her so much, but I'm constantly worried about either making her sick or me getting sick from her. Like this cold. What if she gets it? It could hurt her."

Kathleen remains silent, then says, "Tell me about the education you received prior to adopting your girls."

Eddie accurately explains the transmission of HIV and about opportunistic infections being more severe for HIV-positive children.

"Yes, that's true. But there are ways to protect her as well. Washing your hands frequently, using hand sanitizer, wearing disposable masks for your cold, for example. Plus, I know you pay attention, Eddie. If Cassie gets sick, you're going to get her evaluated quickly." Kathleen states, "In terms of you—did you have an open wound on your hand when you came in contact with Cassie's blood?"

"No. I'd just feel better if I knew for sure."

"I can order the test, if you'd like. How are things going for you and Bill?"

Eddie wipes his nose with a tissue. "We're doing pretty good." He sighs. "Cassie came up to me and started to hump my leg. At first I was shocked and repulsed. Then, I figured out this little girl must have been sexually abused. I had her stop and told her the behavior was not okay. I loved her, but we showed our love in other ways."

Kathleen nods before adding, "That must have been a difficult day for you. But you said the right things. You are teaching her appropriate boundaries, and focusing on behavior and not her as a person. She must have endured significant trauma . . . ."

Eddie went on to tell Kathleen he had gotten Cassie into therapy and "stuff was coming out." He shakes his head. "They didn't tell us about this part. Maybe the caseworker didn't know. I wish we'd known. I mean, we would have still adopted her. It is just harder than I thought it was going to be. Thank God for Bill." He quickly looks at Kathleen as if wanting to know whether she is okay with him being a sexual minority parent.

Kathleen grins. "I'm glad. Partner support means everything when there is a transition in the household like bringing home a child." They continue to talk about trauma-informed parenting and his support from Bill. Kathleen validates and praises Eddie for his parenting style and his hard work at raising the two girls. Eddie describes how he and Bill have become creative in getting Cassie to adhere to her antiretroviral regimen that treats her HIV. He becomes animated when he describes taking "the girls" out for ice cream after school as a treat.

Kathleen assesses his social support and judges him to have good intimate support from his husband, Bill, and his extended network of friends. Subsequent follow-up reveals a negative HIV test for Eddie.

□ □ □ □

CASE STUDY 3: ELIZABETH

Elizabeth is a 40-year-old single parent to a newly adopted 4-year-old daughter. From the time she was a young girl and as an only child, Elizabeth knew she wanted children in her life. Assuming she would have a family by the time she was 35, Elizabeth's career success seemed to outpace her personal goal of marriage and children. Finally, at the age of 38, Elizabeth started plans to adopt through the child welfare system. As the process unfolded, Elizabeth's anticipation grew. She worked with the Department of Child Services (DCS) caseworker and communicated that probably an older child might be a better match for her, given her busy career as the owner of a CPA accounting firm.

A 3-1/2-year-old little girl, Maria, had been removed from her mother's home due to severe neglect and had been with a foster family for 6 months. Prior to being removed from the home, the child was found foraging in the trash for food; however, she has thrived since being placed with a stable foster family. Events moved quickly from there, with Elizabeth being "matched" with Maria and spending increasing amounts of time with her. The mother and father terminated parental rights as both were fighting long-standing charges of drug possession (heroin). The foster mother's reports indicated that Maria, who had no siblings, wanted a permanent home and spoke positively about the time she spent with Elizabeth.

Elizabeth presents to Katy, her family nurse practitioner, requesting a health statement be completed as part of her home study process. Given how much she has enjoyed Maria's company, Elizabeth expects a smooth transition to single parenting and that her life will be fuller and richer as a mother. Elizabeth's affect is bright and other than mild hypertension, which is controlled with hydrochlorothiazide, Katy assesses Elizabeth as in good health. She is confident that Elizabeth is physically and emotionally ready to adopt Maria.

Two months later, Elizabeth returns to Katy's office for presenting complaints of new onset migraine headaches, a 10-pound weight gain, and irritability. Elizabeth's blood pressure is 140/85; weight is 150 pounds (BMI = 28.4). Katy sits down with Elizabeth to discuss how she is feeling. At that time, Elizabeth discloses how she is not sleeping because Maria is insisting on coming into her bed at night. Her daughter is also hoarding food, which Elizabeth finds all over her room, sometimes moldy, and has to be dragged into the day care, which upsets and embarrasses Elizabeth. She then bursts into tears and discloses how the little girl, "doesn't feel like my child. I feel like there is something really wrong with me. Who feels this way? I don't understand—we were bonding *before* I adopted her!"

Elizabeth also admits to work-related problems, being distracted with little motivation to perform well. She believes others in her office have noticed, and she is concerned about her employees who are questioning her stability. She states she is terrified that she has made a huge mistake by adopting Maria. Elizabeth reports her mother was against the adoption, and she has few friends to confide in. She feels she is in crisis with no options and has even considered placing Maria back into the foster care system.

APN Next Steps

Because Katy is an adoption-informed caregiver, she knows the following: Elizabeth is in crisis and may be struggling with parental postadoption depression (PAD). Her patient identified several PAD risk factors: high expectations that did not match the reality of parenting (Foli, 2010), a lack of preparation in understanding the behaviors of children who have experienced trauma, and a lack of social support. While Katy understands she needs to ensure there are no physical changes that would account for Elizabeth's increased blood pressure, headaches, and weight gain, she plans to first screen Elizabeth for depressive symptoms. Katy uses the Patient Health Questionnaire-2 (PHQ-2; Kroenke, Spitzer, & Williams, 2003), a 2-item screening scale. The screen is positive, and Katy understands that this is not a definitive diagnosis of depression; however, a referral to a mental health professional who understands the dynamics of adoption is warranted.

She provides emotional support to Elizabeth by listening, and with congruent verbal and nonverbal communication. Katy reinforces Elizabeth's willingness to share her thoughts and feelings, stating "Today you're identifying and sharing many of your fears. For many adoptive parents, time is needed to bond with their children. Thank you for trusting me." She shares with her patient that PAD is real and faced by many adoptive parents, that she is in a vulnerable transition period and that by strengthening her own functioning, she will be helping Maria. Katy further begins to educate Elizabeth on how Maria's behaviors may stem from past trauma, but there are ways that Elizabeth can help Maria to feel safe, capable, and loved.

Katy refers Elizabeth to an adoption support group in the community, as well as online support groups, prescribes an antidepressant medication, and a list of credible books to help her understand Maria's symptoms of traumatic stress (see Recommended Reading, e.g., *Adopting the Hurt Child; Parenting the Hurt Child* [Keck & Kupecky]). She also recommends that Elizabeth contact the caseworker to ensure that she has been fully informed of what Maria has experienced. She encourages Elizabeth to find play activities that both Maria and she enjoy, such as giving each other manicures, or scrap-booking and helping Maria make a developmentally appropriate "life book" that tells her story.

Four weeks later, Elizabeth returns to see Katy. Her affect is improved and her weight and blood pressure have stabilized. She has experienced only one headache in the past 4 weeks and the pain was relieved by over-the-counter medication. An antidepressant medication is helping to reduce her depressive symptoms. Elizabeth is cautiously optimistic and confides she now realizes how unprepared she was to adopt Maria, but quickly adds that she is so glad that she did. Elizabeth has also reached out to her mother, and they are talking about the experiences of being a single parent.

Elizabeth and Maria have been shopping together and have "spa days" at home where they give each other facials and watch Disney movies together. After reading some of the literature, Elizabeth purchased a sleeping bag for Maria and told her she could sleep in her room if she became scared at night. She leaves a nightlight on in Maria's room and in the hallway to her room, in case Maria wakes up frightened. Maria is also allowed to bring a sandwich bag with a snack in it at night so she does not have to worry about waking up hungry.

Elizabeth is seeing an adoption-competent counselor who helped her understand how there was transference of feelings between Maria and herself. Elizabeth's parents had divorced when she was 5 years old; Maria's fears had rekindled Elizabeth's memories of feeling abandoned and unsafe. She also reports less distractibility at work, and Maria walks into day care without hesitating now. Katy reinforces Elizabeth's problem-solving skills and her perseverance, again finding the strengths in the midst of Elizabeth's crisis.

Katy understands that although the parent, Elizabeth, presented with physical, cognitive, and emotional issues, Katy needed to understand these unique family dynamics. By being adoption-informed, she was able to provide support for this new parent and her vulnerable child so that they could commence with the business of connecting as a family.

□ □ □ □

CASE STUDY 4: THE JOHNSONS

Minda and Seth Johnson, both 26 years old, had always planned to build their family through adoption. Their deep-rooted fundamentalist faith has helped shape their individual identities and their roles within the marriage. The couple has decided to leave their future in God's hands and prayed for direction of how and when a child would come into their lives. Active in their church, Minda has received news from one of the ladies that a young woman has become pregnant and is considering placing the baby. She seeks guidance from their pastor, who believes that the couple would make good parents and encourages them to pursue this adoption. Minda meets with Kallie, the young woman, and they "hit it off" immediately. The birth father, also very young, agrees that the timing of having a child is wrong for him, and he supports placing the child with parents who could give the baby what is needed for a good life.

Minda and Seth decide there is no need for an adoption agency to be involved and arrange for the town's attorney to finalize the adoption when the time comes. They are able to arrange for a home study by a local social worker and complete the state guidelines to be able to adopt. They feel guided to this path and trust events will transpire as they are supposed to.

Kallie has an uneventful pregnancy, and Minda accompanies her to each prenatal check-up. She and Seth provide living expenses, helping Kallie with her food and letting her stay in a spare bedroom while she is pregnant. Kallie encourages Minda to select a name for the baby, and Minda and Seth decide upon Rachel. When Kallie delivers the baby girl, Minda is there in the delivery room. Social services are notified, and the nurses are aware of the adoption plan.

Kallie asks to hold the baby upon birth, and Minda knows when she sees them bond that something has changed. She knows then that Kallie is not going to relinquish Rachel to her. Kallie asks Minda to leave the room, adding, "I don't think I can go through with this. I just can't give her up." Minda feels as if she is going to be sick and steps into the hallway. She leaves the hospital as soon as she can, and drives home to call Seth, who is at work.

Two months later, Minda is due for her annual physical. Her family nurse practitioner, Lauren, sees Minda and notes that she has lost 10 pounds, looks fatigued, and has a flat affect. Her complete blood count indicates a low hemoglobin level and high white blood cell count.

APN Next Steps

Lauren begins the physical examination and asks Minda how she is feeling. Minda replies, "Fine," in a monotone voice. She added, "I cut my hair and don't always wear skirts anymore. I feel more free, you know?"

Lauren pauses, but Minda does not say anything further. She begins to discuss Minda's diet and shares that Minda's BMI of 18 is low. Minda shrugs her shoulders, saying, "I'm just not hungry."

Lauren stands beside Minda and continues with the examination of her ears, nose, and throat. Minda complains of fatigue, difficulty swallowing, and Lauren notes white spots on the back of her mouth and soft palate. Lauren obtains a swab specimen from Minda's throat and performs a rapid antigen test. The results are positive for strep throat. She hands Minda a prescription for an antibiotic and states, "I feel as if there's something else going on."

Minda swallows, winces, and says, "Well, I thought I'd be a mother by now."

Lauren's confused, and says, "You thought you would be a mother . . ."

Minda nods and becomes tearful. She relates what happened with Kallie and the baby. She adds that since that time, she has rejected her church, begun to wear pants instead of skirts, and cut her hair as signs of her loss of faith. Lauren listens, restates, and summarizes what Minda tells her.

As an adoption-competent APN, Lauren knows that what Minda has experienced has caused her to grieve someone invisible to society. She assesses Minda's sleep and diet, as well as her social support network, especially since she has become estranged from her church. Minda reports experiencing anorexia, fatigue, and insomnia. She rarely goes out of the house and because of her choice not to attend church, she has lost an important support network. After noting

Minda's diet (lots of hot tea and toast), Lauren is convinced her low hemoglobin is related to her dietary intake.

Lauren explains to Minda that she is grieving a loss, and that it is okay to feel sad, angry, confused, and want to reject those things she feels somehow betrayed her. Minda confides that she has been unable to talk about the loss and feels as if she was duped, yet understands Kallie's reasons for wanting to keep the baby. She understands now that both she and Kallie should have received preparation and counseling throughout the months leading up to birth so that they would be prepared, no matter what the final outcome was. Lauren educates Minda that Kallie's decision was about Kallie and the baby, and not about Minda and Seth. She validates Minda's feelings of anger, regret, loss, and sadness. Lauren also offers information about reputable online adoption support groups whose members could relate to Minda's loss. She shares resources about grief and loss with Minda and arranges to see her again in 8 weeks to recheck hemoglobin levels. However, she instructs Minda to watch for fever, dehydration, or worsening symptoms of her strep throat and to call the office or emergency department after hours if that were to happen. She also refers Minda to a dietitian for instructions on improving her diet and discusses slow-release iron supplements.

Follow-Up

Minda's strep throat has resolved, and she returns for a follow-up appointment for nutritional status. Emily reviews the electronic medical record and notes that the laboratory reports are normal, the patient has gained 4 pounds, and she looks more rested. Her affect is overall sad, but she is able to smile appropriately throughout the interaction. Minda believes that adoption may still work for her and Seth, but she needs some time. Her feelings for Kallie have also softened with an increased empathy toward how difficult the decision to relinquish a child must be. She and Seth have returned to their pastor to discuss their loss and are receiving support through lay parishioners trained in counseling.

APNS' CARE OF ADOPTIVE PARENTS

Caring for the needs of adoptive parents, as with other members of the triad, is contingent upon the experiences of the parents and child.

TABLE 4.1   *Adoptive Parents: What to Look for and What to Do*

Adoptive Parents

What to Look for (Assessment):

☐ Assess physical condition when asked to sign medical report attesting to the prospective parent's health status.

☐ Monitor for signs of postadoption depression as well as grief (especially from failed adoptions) and other mood disorders in adoptive parents.

☐ Assess social support for mothers and fathers.

☐ Tease out physical complaints that may be related to psychosocial needs.

☐ Assess accuracy of information related to the child's needs that was relayed prior to adoption.

☐ Assess adequacy of postadoption services.

☐ Monitor for signs of adoption dissolution or disruption.

☐ Assess for microaggressions against sexual minority parents.

What to Do (Management):

☐ Support efforts to breastfeed when appropriate.

☐ Provide psychosocial support and therapeutic communication before and after placement.

☐ Support open adoption plans unless contraindicated for the safety and well-being of the child.

☐ Immediately report rehoming or unregulated custody transfers.

☐ Refer adoptive parent to needed resources to strengthen parenting role.

☐ Ensure the parent is providing a safe and nurturing environment for the child.

The heterogeneity of adoptive parents is growing with more sexual minority parents being included. APNs are cautioned to avoid dismissal of the needs of parents based on demographics alone (higher incomes, educational levels, etc.) and to appreciate the complexities of integrating a child into a family unit and the transition faced once a child is place into the home (Table 4.1).

CHAPTER HIGHLIGHTS

☐ Adoptive parents, while heterogeneous, are more likely to be older, more educated, and have higher incomes than birth parents.

☐ Adoptive parents' primary motivations to adopt include providing a permanent home for a child and expanding their family.

☐ The adoption process consists of preadoption preparation and training, waiting for a referral and placement of a child, and postplacement integration of the child into the family.

☐ Sexual minority parents have more contact with birth parents and report positive experiences with them. However, some same-sex parents report more parenting stress.

☐ Postadoption services are necessary for successful placement of the child.

☐ The National Child Traumatic Stress Network offers a wide range of resources for APNs to access and share with patients.

☐ Parental attachment to the child is one key factor to successful placement.

☐ Rehoming, or unregulated custody transfer, is a deplorable act that places the child in grave danger.

☐ Parental postadoption depression (PAD) should be screened for by APNs to optimize parental functioning and avoid negative outcomes for the child.

Questions for Reflection

Following are a few questions to reflect upon. You can use these to start a journal for yourself or in a classroom discussion with peers and the instructor.

1. When you consider adoptive parents, do you tend to generalize them into a demographic profile of older, more educated, higher socioeconomic status, and White? Do you see them as part of a dominant culture? Is this a balanced appraisal? Why or why not?

2. When you see a conspicuous family (transracial), what thoughts do you have? Is it fair to the child to be raised by parents of a different ethnicity and race? What would mitigate the differences between child and parent?

3. Do you see different-sex and same-sex adoptive parents as equally capable of raising healthy, happy children? Why or why not?

4. As an APN, how would you approach adoptive parents who refuse to prepare for a child because of a previously failed adoption? What rationale would you offer to them that preparation is needed? How would you address their loss and grief?

5. What case study spoke to you the most? Why? What personal and professional feelings were evoked within you?

References

American Academy of Family Physicians. (2016). Family physicians supporting breastfeeding: A position paper (adoptive breastfeeding). Retrieved from www.aafp.org/about/policies/all/breastfeeding-support.html

American Academy of Pediatrics. (2005). Breastfeeding and the use of human milk. *Pediatrics, 115*(2), 496–506.

Beck, C. T. (1996a). Postpartum depressed mothers' experiences interacting with their children. *Nursing Research, 45,* 98–104.

Beck, C. T. (1996b). Predictors of postpartum depression: A meta-analysis. *Nursing Research, 45,* 297–303.

Beck, C. T. (1998). A checklist to identify women at risk for developing postpartum depression. *Journal of Obstetric, Gynecologic, and Neonatal Nursing, 27*(1), 39–46.

Beck, C. T. (2002a). Revision of the Postpartum Depression Predictors Inventory. *Journal of Obstetric, Gynecologic, and Neonatal Nursing, 31*(4), 394–402.

Beck, C. T. (2002b). Theoretical perspectives of postpartum depression. *MCN: The American Journal of Maternal Child Nursing, 27,* 282–287.

Beck, C. T., Records, K., & Rice, M. (2006). Further development of the Postpartum Depression Predictors Inventory-Revised. *Journal of Obstetric, Gynecologic, and Neonatal Nursing, 35*(6), 735–745.

Bond, J. (1995). Post-adoption depression syndrome. *Roots and Wings Adoption Magazine, Spring.*

Bos, H. M. W., Knox, J. R., van Rijin-van Gelderen, L., & Gartrell, N. K. (2016). Same-sex and different-sex parent households and child health outcomes: Findings from the National Survey of Children's Health. *Journal of Behavioral and Developmental Pediatrics, 37*(3), 179–187.

Brodinsky, D. (2015). *The modern adoptive families study.* New York, NY: The Donaldson Adoption Institute.

Brodinsky, D. M., & Goldberg, A. E. (2016a). Contact with birth family in adoptive families headed by lesbian, gay, and heterosexual parents. *Children and Youth Services Review, 62,* 9–17. doi:10.1016/j.childyouth.2016.01.014

Brodinsky, D. M., & Goldberg, A. E. (2016b). *Practice guidelines supporting open adoption in families headed by lesbian and gay male parents: Lessons learned from the Modern Adoptive Family study.* Donaldson Adoption Institute. Retrieved from adoptioninstitute.org/wordpress/wp-content/

uploads/2016/05/DAI_MAFReport2.pdf?mc_cid=aeb5e66449&mc_eid=06d431f287

Bureau of Consular Affairs, U.S. State Department. (2016). Intercountry adoption: Universal Accreditation Act of 2012. Retrieved from https://travel.state.gov/content/adoptionsabroad/en/hague-convention/agency-accreditation/universal-accreditation-act-of-2012.html

Cherguit, J., Burns, J., Pettle, S., & Tasker, F. (2013) Lesbian co-mothers' experiences of maternity healthcare services. *Journal of Advanced Nursing, 69*(6), 1269–1278. doi:10.1111/j.1365-2648.2012.06115.x

Child Welfare Information Gateway. (2012). Adoption disruption and dissolution. Washington, DC: U.S. Department of Health and Human Services, Children's Bureau. Retrieved from www.childwelfare.gov/pubPDFs/s_disrup.pdf

Child Welfare Information Gateway. (2015). The adoption home study process. Washington, DC: U.S. Department of Health and Human Services, Children's Bureau. Retrieved from www.childwelfare.gov/pubpdfs/f_homstu.pdf

Dean, C., Dean, N. R., White, A., & Liu, W. Z. (1995). An adoption study comparing the prevalence of psychiatric illness in women who have adoptive and natural children compared with women who have adoptive children only. *Journal of Affective Disorders, 34*, 55–60.

Evan B. Donaldson Institute, North American Council on Adoptable Children, & Adoption Support and Preservation. (2012). *The vital role of adoption subsidies increasing permanency and improving children' lives (while saving states money)*. New York, NY: Author.

Fields, E. S., Meuchel, J. M., Jaffe, C. J., Jha, M. & Payne, J. L. (2010). Post adoption depression. *Erratum to Archives of Women's Mental Health, 13*, 147–151. doi:10.1007/s00737-009-0137-7

Foli, K. J. (2010). Depression in adoptive parents: A model of understanding through grounded theory. *Western Journal of Nursing Research, 32*, 379–400. doi:10.1177/0193945909351299

Foli, K. J., South, S. C., & Lim, E. (2012a). Rates and predictors of depression in adoptive mothers: Moving toward theory. *Advances in Nursing Science, 35*(1), 51–63. doi:10.1097/ANS.0b013e318244553e

Foli, K. J. South, S. C., Lim, E., & Hebdon, M. (2012b). Depression in adoptive fathers: An exploratory mixed methods study. *Psychology of Men & Masculinity*. doi:10.1037/a0030482

Foli, K. J., South, S. C., Lim, E., & Hebdon, M. (2016a). Longitudinal course of risk for parental post-adoption depression using the postpartum depression predictors inventory-revised. *Journal of Obstetric, Gynecologic, and Neonatal Nursing, 45*, 210–226, doi:org/10.1016/j.jogn.2015.12.011

Foli, K. J., South, S. C., Lim, E., & Jarnecke, A. (2016b). Post-adoption depression: Parental classes of depressive symptoms across time. *Journal of Affective Disorders, 200*, 293–302. doi:10.1016/j.jad.2016.01.049

Foli, K. J., & Thompson, J. R. (2004). *The post-adoption blues: Overcoming the unforeseen challenges of adoption.* Emmaus, PA: Rodale.

Fontenot, H. B. (2007). Transition and adaptation to adoptive motherhood. *Journal of the Obstetric, Gynecologic, and Neonatal Nursing, 36*, 175–182. doi:10.1111/J.1552-6909.2007.00134.x

Gair, S. (1999). Distress and depression in new motherhood: Research with adoptive mothers highlights important contributing factors. *Child and Family Social Work, 4*, 55–66.

Gates, G. J. (2013). *LGBT parenting in the United States* (pp. 1–6). Los Angeles, CA: The Williams Institute.

Gates, G. (2014). *LGB families and relationships: Analysis of the 2013 National Health Interview Survey.* Los Angeles, CA: The Williams Institute.

Gavin, N. I., Gaynes, B. N., Lohr, K. N., Meltzer-Brody, S., Gartlehner, G., & Swinson, T. (2005). Perinatal depression: A systematic review of prevalence and incidence. *Obstetrics and Gynecology, 106*, 1071–1083.

Goldberg, A. E., & Smith, J. Z. (2011). Stigma, social context, and mental health: Lesbian and gay couples across the transition to adoptive parenthood. *Journal of Counseling Psychology, 58*(1), 139–150. doi:10.1037/a0021684

Government Accountability Office. (2015). *Steps have been taken to address unregulated custody transfers of adopted children.* New York, NY: Author.

Hanna, M. D., & McRoy, R. G. (2011). Innovative practice approaches to matching in adoption. *Journal of Public Child Welfare, 5*(1), 45–66. doi:10.1080/15548732.2011.542722

James, A. (2009). *Brothers and sisters in adoption: Helping children navigate relationships when new kids join the family.* Indianapolis, IN: Perspectives Press.

Jennings, S., Mellish, L., Tasker, F., Lamb, M., & Golombok, S. (2014). Why adoption? Gay, lesbian, and heterosexual adoptive parents' reproductive experiences and reasons for adoption. *Adoption Quarterly, 17*(3), 205–226. doi:10.1080/10926755.2014.891549

Jones, J. (2009). *Who adopts? Characteristics of women and men who have adopted children.* NCHS Data Brief, No 12. Hyattsville, MD: National Center for Health Statistics.

Kennedy, H., Beck, C.T., & Driscoll, J. (2002). A light in the fog: Caring for women with postpartum depression. *Journal of Midwifery & Women's Health, 47,* 318–330.

Kroenke, K., Spitzer, R.L., Williams, J.B. (2003). The patient health questionnaire-2: Validity of a two item depression screener. *Medical Care, 41,* 1284–1294.

La Leche League International. (2008–2016). Can I breastfeed my adopted baby? Retrieved from www.lalecheleague.org/faq/adopt.html

McKay, K., & Ross, L.E. (2009). The transition to adoptive parenthood: A pilot study of parents adopting in Ontario, Canada. *Children and Youth Services Review, 32,* 604–610. doi:10.1016/j.childyouth.2009.12.007

McKay, K., Ross, L. E., & Goldberg, A. E. (2010). Adaptation to parenthood during the post-adoption period: A review of the literature. *Adoption Quarterly, 13,* 125–144. doi:10.1080/10926755.2010.481040

Mott, S. L., Schiller, C. E., Richards, J. G., O'Hara, M. W., & Stuart, S. (2011). Depression and anxiety among postpartum and adoptive mothers. *Archives of Women's Mental Health. 14,* 335–343. doi:10.1007/s00737-011-0227-1

National Child Traumatic Stress Network. (2015). The NCTSN mission and vision. Retrieved from www.nctsn.org/about-us/mission-and-vision

O'Hara, M. S., & Swain, A. M. (1996). Rates and risk of postpartum depression: A meta-analysis. *International Review of Psychiatry, 8,* 37–54.

Paulson, J. F., & Bazemore, S. D. (2010). Prenatal and postpartum depression in fathers and its association with maternal depression. *Journal of the American Medical Association, 303*(19), 1961–1969.

Pemberton, C.K., Neiderhiser, J.M., Leve, L.D., Natsuaki, M.N., Shaw, D.S., Reiss, D., Ge, X. (2010). Influence of parental depressive symptoms on adopted toddler behaviors: An emerging developmental cascade of genetic and environmental effects. *Developmental Psychopathology, 22,* 803–818. doi:10.1017/S09545794100004774

Radloff, L. S. (1977). The CES-D scale: A self-report depression scale for research in the general population. *Applied Psychological Measurement, 1*(3), 385–401.

Rolock, N. (2015). Post-permanency continuity: What happens after adoption and guardianship from foster care? *Journal of Public Child Welfare, 9*, 153–173. doi:10.1080/15548732.2015.1021986

Rykkje, L. (2007). Intercountry adoption and nursing care. *Scandinavian Journal of Caring Sciences, 21*(4), 507–514.

Senecky, Y., Hanoch, A., Inbar, D., Horesh, N., Diamond, G., Bergman, Y. S., & Apte, A. (2009). Post-adoption depression among adoptive mothers. *Journal of Affective Disorders, 115*, 62–68.

Smith, S. L. (2010). *Keeping the promise: The critical need for post-adoption services to enable children and families to succeed.* New York, NY: Donaldson Adoption Institute. Retrieved from adoptioninstitute.org/research/2010_10_promises.php

Smith, S. L. (2013). *A family for life: The vital need to achieve permanency for children in care.* New York, NY: Donaldson Adoption Institute. Retrieved from adoptioninstitute.org/research/2013_04_FamilyForLife.php.

Smith, S. L. (2014). *Supporting and preserving adoptive families: Profiles of publicly funded post-adoption services.* New York, NY: The Donaldson Institute.

South, S. C., Foli, K. J., & Lim, E. (2012). Predictors of relationship satisfaction in adoptive mothers. *Journal of Social and Personal Relationships, 30*(5), 545–563. doi:10.1177/0265407512462681

Tully, E.C., Iacono, W.G., McGue, M. (2008). An adoption study of parental depression as an environmental liability for adolescent depression and childhood disruptive disorders. *The American Journal of Psychiatry, 165*, 1148–1154.

Twohey, M. (2013). Reuters Investigates: Americans use the Internet to abandon children adopted from overseas. Retrieved from www.reuters.com/investigates/adoption/#article/part1/sidebar/emails/email/218

U.S. Census Bureau. (2010). 2010 Census urban and rural classification and urban area criteria: Urban, urbanized area, urban cluster, and rural population, 2010 and 2000: United States. Retrieved from www.census.gov/geo/reference/ua/urban-rural-2010.html

Vandivere, S., Malm, K., & Radel, L. (2009). *Adoption USA: A chartbook based on the 2007 National Survey of Adoptive Parents.* Washington, DC: The U.S. Department of Health and Human Services, Office of the Assistant Secretary for Planning and Evaluation.

Vesga-Lopez, O., Blanco, C., Keyes, K., Olfson, M., Grant, B. F., & Hasin, D.S. (2008). Psychiatric disorders in pregnant and postpartum women in the United States. *Archives of General Psychiatry, 65*, 805–815.

Wright, G. (2011). Intensive support for adoptive families living in rural areas. *White Paper Series, 1*(105). Kinship Center Education Institute.

Wydra, M., O'Brien, K. M., & Merson, E. S. (2012). In their own words: Adopted persons' experiences of adoption disclosure and discussion in their families. *Journal of Family Social Work, 15*(1), 62–77. doi:10.1080/1052 2158.2012.642616

5

The Child/Adult Who Is Adopted

□ □ □ □

PURPOSE OF THE CHAPTER

This chapter is an expansion of Chapter 2, which focused on adopted children from a pediatric health care perspective. Broader issues are covered in this chapter, including maltreatment of children, educational and social issues, and transracial adoption. Outcomes of children adopted by same-sex individuals are also discussed. The adoption community emphasizes that adoption is not a one-time occurrence or transaction; rather it is a "lifelong transformation" (Donaldson Adoption Institute, 2016). This is especially true for those individuals who are adopted. Each narrative is unique and based on many factors: the type of adoption (domestic private, public welfare/foster care, and intercountry), the age of the child at adoption, the experiences of the individual before being adopted (e.g., exposure to drugs and alcohol in utero, institutional care, maltreatment), and the competency of the adoptive parents (e.g., sensitivity to transracial and cultural identity, knowledge and commitment to addressing trauma-born behaviors, expectations).

We review four cases that bring to advanced practice nurses' (APNs) attention how health care needs may be in direct connection with the adoption process, as is the case for medically compromised intercountry-adopted children and those whose health-related behaviors emanate from being an adopted person. From a young boy, adopted from Ethiopia, to a 12-year-old girl, who has begun acting out, to a transracially adopted college student, to, finally, a successful professional who engages in high-risk behaviors, we describe the connections between health care–driven needs of adopted persons and the interventions to support optimal health and well-being.

Learning Objectives

At the completion of the chapter, the reader will be able to:

1. Identify demographic characteristics of adopted children and adults
2. Synthesize the potential and known links among psychological issues, adverse childhood experiences, and physical diseases in adopted persons
3. Appreciate the historical context of sealed or closed adoption records and current trends in select states that are opening birth records to adopted persons
4. Be able to counsel children and adolescents with the W.I.S.E. Up! Tool in dialoguing with individuals about being adopted
5. Increase cultural sensitivity to the orientation of transracially adopted individuals
6. Relate current evidence on child outcomes of same-sex parents
7. Argue the pros and cons of genetic testing for adopted persons

OVERVIEW OF ADOPTED CHILDREN

The majority of adopted children are from racial and ethnic minorities: 62% of children who are adopted are of minority status (non-Hispanic Black: 23%; non-Hispanic Asian: 15%; Hispanic: 15%; and other non-Hispanic: 9%) compared with 44% of all U.S. children (Vandivere, Malm, & Radel, 2009). Adopted children are also more likely to live in homes with parents who have attended college and have higher incomes than nonadopted children (Bramlett, Radel, & Blumberg, 2007).

Access to Medical Information

There are two aspects to openness in adoption. First, the sealing of birth certificates at the time of birth, thereby denying access to adopted persons to their original birth certificates. And second, the movement toward some sort of contact with birth parents after parental rights have been terminated. Historically, closed adoptions were the norm with original birth certificates being sealed and the child being given a new name. As the Maternal–Child Health Interdivisional Council of Colorado League for Nursing (1961) stated,

The records shall be kept confidential and shall be sealed and opened only for inspection upon the order of the court for good cause.

In the case of adoption of any person the state registrar, upon receipt of a certified copy of the adoption decree or a report from the court having decreed the adoption, shall prepare a birth certificate in the new name of the adopted person and shall seal and file the original certificate of birth with the certified copy of the adoption decree or report of the court, and all other papers pertaining to the old certificate shall be attached thereto.

As discussed in the history of adoption in Chapter 1, confidential or closed adoptions are much less common today. Both closed and open adoptions have implications for the APN. As legislation is introduced to unseal birth certificates, the APN needs to be aware of what medical information is available or unavailable to individuals who are adopted. Vigilance in screenings and health promotion activities should be reflected in the care of adopted persons.

Genetic Testing

Aspects of genetic testing within the adoption context are important to explain. These aspects pertain to who is requesting the testing and for what purposes. In the first instance, the testing may be done before the decision to adopt a specific child, and to determine whether the adoption will proceed, either during pregnancy or immediately after birth. The second genetic testing is requested by the adopted individual, usually an adult, to learn more about his or her ancestry and health background, and possibly toward efforts of reunification.

Importantly, genetic testing of adopted individuals has been discussed at increasing rates. In response to the growing requests from prospective adoptive parents and adoption agencies, the American Society of Human Genetics (ASHG) Social Issues Committee and the American College of Medical Genetics (ACMG) Social, Ethical, and Legal Issues Committee (2000) issued a statement specific to testing in the context of adoption. The first recommendation states:

All genetic testing of newborns and children in the adoption process should be consistent with the tests performed on all children of a similar age for the purposes of diagnosis or of identifying appropriate prevention strategies.

The rationales for this recommendation are that (a) testing results may make adoption more difficult for the infant/child; (b) the infant/child may be treated differently by the parents, and (c) a child who is adopted should be treated as any biological child in the family; genetic testing should be in the best interest of the child (ASHG & ACMG, 2000). Others argue that current practices in pre-adoptive genetic testing are too restrictive and counter that adoptive parents need to know about genetic factors and thus would be able to provide for the child in a more informed way—a type of matching of parent and child. The argument also asserts that genetic testing falls under medical disclosures to adoptive parents during the adoption process and could potentially make it easier to place special needs children (Taylor, 2008).

With the Human Genome Project announcement that the entire genetic code for one individual had been mapped, coupled with the issue of access to medical histories, many adopted individuals are considering genomic testing to determine risks for certain diseases. Direct-to-consumer (DTC) genetic testing is becoming more prevalent and, although a comprehensive discussion is beyond the scope of this book, it is important for the APN to understand the DTC testing, as well as the emergence of genetics/genomics nursing (American Nurses Association [ANA] & The International Society of Nurses in Genetics, 2016). This specialty area focuses on the impact of genetic/genomic information on the health and well-being of individuals and will be important resources for adopted individuals who either have or seek such information.

Proprietary companies that provide genetic testing, such as 23andMe (2015), which received approval from the FDA in February 2015 for the Bloom syndrome carrier genetic test, have tried previously to offer full genetic testing directly to individuals. Creating a DNA database specific to children adopted from Korea is the goal of 325Kamra, a nonprofit organization designed to explore the biological heritage of Korea and potentially use the database as a method to reunite adopted persons with birth families (325Kamra, 2016). Individuals without access to medical records have argued these genetic tests are needed so that they can understand health care risks and genetic predispositions.

Transracial Adoption

Transracial adoption—parents and children of different races and ethnicities—has a history of controversy that continues to stimulate lively discussions in the adoption world about race, culture, and identity. Transracial/transethnic adoptions may be mixtures of White, Black, Asian, Native American, and Hispanic. Based on data from the National Survey of Adoptive Parents (NSAP), the National Center for Marriage and Family Research tabulated transracial adoptions by adoption type (see Figure 5.1). Almost 40% of all adoptions are transracial, with nearly 84% of intercountry adoptions being transracial (Ela, 2011). Private domestic adoptions account for the smallest number of transracial adoptions at 21.3% (Ela, 2011). Lesbian and gay couples are more likely than heterosexual couples to adopt transracially and are themselves more likely to be interracial (Farr & Patterson, 2009). For members of transracial adoption triads, the lifelong impact of adoption becomes even more important as the child grows, questions his or her identity, and resolves issues of culture, class, and race.

I myself am a part of a transracial adoption triad, an adoptive mother to a daughter who came to us from India at 5.5 months. We have experienced behaviors from health care professionals who are not used to conspicuous families. When I take her to her primary care visits, I often receive messages from providers who seek

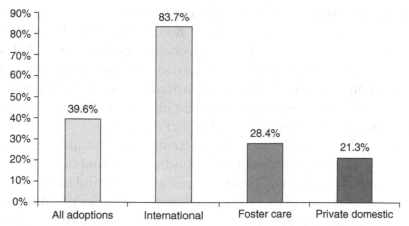

FIGURE 5.1   *Percentage of adoptions that are transracial, by adoption type.*
Source: Ela (2011). Reprinted by permission of the National Center for Family and Marriage Research.

excessive verification that I am her mother and excessive verification of the information I extend regarding her health. When we are in public, folks used to stare at us and, over the years, I have become desensitized to them. When I was discussing this with an adoption professional, I emphasized how the stares, the looks because we were conspicuous, did not matter to me. "Aahh," the adoption professional said to me, "But it might matter to her." This was my epiphany, one that I am grateful for. It has made me sensitive to what she thinks, needs, and wants: how she makes sense of the conspicuousness of our family and her own identity and place in the world.

Children of Same-Sex Parents

In the 2000 census, 10% of same-sex couples with children reported raising adopted children (Brodinsky, 2015). Empirically, outcomes for children (including adopted children) raised by sexual minority parents have been the focus of several studies. Farr, Crain, Oakley, Cashen, and Garber (2016) found that, despite evidence of microaggressions toward children with same-sex parents, children demonstrated resilience and reported positive conceptualizations about their families. In a large sample of children with same-sex parents (which included adopted children), school performance was compared with other family structures (Rosenfeld, 2010). Findings described how children of sexual minority parents were as likely to make progress through school as children of other family structures (Rosenfeld, 2010). However, these findings were challenged by Allen, Pakaluk, and Price (2013) when different comparison and sample groups were used. Compared with traditional married households, children of same-sex parents were statistically less likely to make normal progress through school (Allen, Pakaluk, & Price, 2013).

Research is needed to examine the *contributors* to child outcomes. In a large sample, time spent with children of sexual minority and heterosexual couples was analyzed; researchers found that women, regardless of the sex of the partner, and men in same-sex couples spent more time with the child than did men in heterosexual relationships (Prickett, Marin-Storey, & Crosnoe, 2015). Additional factors that contribute to positive outcomes for all children need to be described, measured, and compared between same-sex and traditional families.

In Chapter 4, we discussed the Modern Adoptive Families (MAF) study (Brodinsky, 2015), a landmark initiative to better understand adopted children who are being raised by sexual minority parents. A summary of current literature and policy recommendations can be found online through the Donaldson Adoption Institute (Brodinsky, 2015). Public opinion, inclusivity, and finding nurturing, safe homes for children have overcome previous barriers and stereotypes of sexual minority parents' suitability to become adoptive parents. Professional organizations such as the American Medical Association, the American Academy of Pediatrics, Child Welfare League of America, and the American Psychological Association have issued statements confirming that sexual orientation should not be a barrier to adoption.

MENTAL HEALTH ISSUES IN ADOPTED CHILDREN AND ADOLESCENTS

The history of adoption research into the psychological aspects of adoption would fill more pages than this chapter will allow. Throughout the past 60 years, there has been tension in the adoption community between meeting the needs of the child versus the needs of the adoptive parents. As adopted children became a focus of study, multiple investigations reported a disproportionate number of adopted individuals having behavioral and mental health issues. Baden and O'Leary Wiley (2007) forward four potential reasons for these findings: (a) studies in the 1960s characterized by the psychodynamic approach emphasized the adoptive parents' potential inability to bond with the children and the adoptees' resentment over being relinquished; (b) in more recent accounts, the experiences before adoption created maladaptive coping strategies (see discussion on adverse childhood experiences [ACEs] that follows); (c) genetic and environmental risk factors from the birth parents contribute to behavioral issues in adopted individuals; and (d) because adoptive parents seek out care for their children in a disproportionate manner, the statistics compiled for adopted children reflect higher numbers of difficulties. A brief review of the literature that focused on *adults* who are adopted, revealed that these individuals may be at increased risks of depression, suicide, anxiety, and substance use disorders (Forster, Foli, Abrahamson, & Richards, 2016).

Another approach to examining the psychological literature and connect findings to clinical practice is along three major categories: identity development, search and reunion, and long-term outcomes (Baden & O'Leary Wiley, 2007). The first is a large body of research that attempts to describe the questions and answers surrounding adoptee's identity: Who am I? Where did I come from? Why was I relinquished? The second area, search and reunion, is viewed either as a normal desire to meet biological parents versus a pathological process linked to dissatisfaction with the adoption. The last, based on studies, long-term outcomes of adopted individuals reflect poorer psychological adjustment; however, the authors also note that interpretation of these results varies across researchers, in some cases with an absence of control for variables that impact such findings (e.g., openness in adoption, preadoption conditions; Baden & O'Leary Wiley, 2007). Threaded through these areas are adopted individuals' attachment and bonding issues; issues of intimacy and abandonment; and behavioral health issues (e.g., depression, substance use). APNs should note the individual experiences of the adopted person, who may or may not present with mental health issues, and management should be guided by a priority of patient safety.

Trauma and Environments of Deprivation

Beginning in 1990, international adoptions from Eastern European nations grew as countries from the former Soviet Union emerged and thousands of orphans residing in institutions became available for adoption. In the subsequent years, the extent of childhood deprivation, maltreatment, and prenatal exposure to alcohol also became apparent. The body of research produced by Teena McGuinness and colleagues describes this population of intercountry-adopted children from Eastern European countries (e.g., McGuinness & Dyer, 2006; McGuinness, McGuinness, & Dyer, 2000; McGuinness & Pallansch, 2007; McGuinness & Robinson, 2011). In a structural equation model, latent variables of risk (birth weight, age at institutionalization, and length of time in orphanage), competence (externalizing behaviors, school, and socialization), and family environment (expressiveness and cohesion) were examined in 105 children adopted from the former Soviet Union. Although previous adverse experiences were reported (e.g., 41% of the birth mothers had abused alcohol), families served as a buffer to the risks and low competency scores (McGuinness, McGuinness, & Dyer, 2000). This sample was followed across time and later reassessed to determine the effects of time: Birth weight was the only risk factor that continued to be associated with problem behavior scores. Aspects of the family environment (buffers to the risks) increased in influence over time (McGuinness & Pallansch, 2007).

Longitudinal studies and cross-sectional studies surrounding inter-country adoption conducted in the 1990s were reviewed by McGuinness and Dyer (2006). Although international adoption has been termed a "natural experiment" (p. 276) in that genetics and environmental influences may be viewed separately, the authors conclude that the study of internationally adopted children is in reality a "multicausal model" (p. 286). Asserting that while adoptive parents continue to influence positive outcomes, certain groups of internationally adopted children remain at risk for poor outcomes, particularly those children adopted from Romania (McGuinness & Dyer, 2006).

If we accept that any child who has transitioned away from his or her birth parents has experienced trauma, then we begin to understand how some adopted individuals circle around and fall into a life of trauma. Understanding trauma is intertwined with understanding ACEs and the subsequent implications for diseases and well-being across the life span. If, as an APN, you are question-ing the link between mental and physical health, the ACE studies provide evidence of the strength of that link. The groundbreaking study conducted by Felitti et al. (1998) revealed that ACE scores of 9,508 individuals in a large health maintenance organization were associated with both mental health and disease states. Twenty-five percent of the participants reported two or more adverse experi-ences. Persons with four or more categories, when compared with those that had no experience, had a 4- to-12-times increased risk for alcoholism, drug abuse, depression, and suicide attempt. Exposure to ACEs was linked to ischemic heart disease, cancer, chronic lung disease, skeletal fractures, and liver disease (Felitti et al., 1998; see Figure 5.2).

In a current study by Fox, Perez, Cass, Baglivio, and Epps (2015), ACEs were divided into nine items creating the childhood adverse

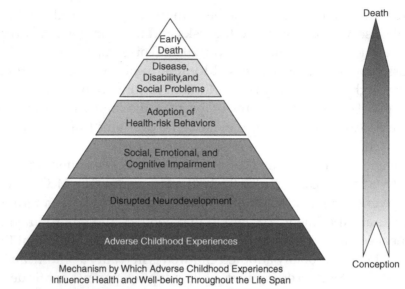

FIGURE 5.2   *The adverse childhood experiences (ACE) pyramid.*
Source: Centers for Disease Control and Prevention (2016).

experiences index: ACE 1: emotional abuse; ACE 2: physical abuse; ACE 3: sexual abuse; ACE 4: emotional neglect; ACE 5: physical neglect; ACE 6: household violence; ACE 7: household substance abuse; ACE 8: household mental illness; and ACE 9: incarcerated household member. Using data on 22,575 juvenile offenders, the researchers found that each additional experience increased the overall risk of becoming a serious, chronic, and violent juvenile offender by 35 (Fox, Perez, Cass, Baglivio, & Epps, 2015). Implications for adopted persons who have experienced ACEs and APNs who are involved in these persons care are evident; the ACE index may be a helpful guide in assessing the adverse experiences of adopted individuals and understanding implications for future health states.

SOCIAL AND EDUCATIONAL ISSUES AND ADOPTION

Adoption disclosures are when adoptive and kinship parents inform their children that they are indeed adopted. These disclosures, which should be developmentally appropriate, occur as soon as possible in the child's life so that the child can begin to craft a narrative and make sense of his or her origins. However, acquaintances and society in general are often curious when they see conspicuous families or discover that an individual is adopted. The Center for Adoption Support and Education (CASE; n.d.) has developed a program for adopted children and persons to use when faced with questions about being part of a nontraditional family. Singer (2010) outlines the background and resources available through CASE, situating the discussion within pediatric nursing. An approach to help adopted children field questions is offered in Exhibit 5.1 (Schoettle, 2000; Singer, 2010).

EXHIBIT 5.1
THE W.I.S.E. UP! TOOL

- ☐ **W:** *Walk away or ignore what you hear.*
- ☐ **I:** *It's private. I do not have to share information with anyone and I can say that appropriately, even to adults.*
- ☐ **S:** *Share something about my adoption story, but I can think carefully about what I want to let others know.*
- ☐ **E:** *Educate others about adoption in general. For example, I can talk about how adoption works today, successful adoptees, and inaccurate information in the media.*

Source: Schoettle (2000).

Offering a tool such as the W.I.S.E. Up! tool as a planned approach will assist the child in becoming empowered and confident. The questions will come regardless. But if the child or adolescent is prepared, he or she can address the queries with responses that will allow the child to protect his or her narrative, educate others, and proactively understand what is in his or her comfort zone to share. This tool, although designed for children who are adopted, can be used by kinship children as well. When asked about their parents or receiving comments about grandparents who are raising them (e.g., "Your mom looks old"), kinship children can prepare responses to include positive messages, such as, "My grandmother is taking care of me now. I know she loves me a lot."

REUNIFICATION, REUNIONS, AND REMEMBERING

Reunifications occur when children are reunified with their birth parents before adoption. In September 2014, 55% of children and adolescents in foster care were identified as having the goal of reunification with their birth parents or caretakers, up from 51% in 2005 (Child Welfare Information Gateway, 2016). Various scales and assessments are used in case planning to determine whether reunification is a viable choice. Being reunified with birth parents may or may not be permanent for the child, especially if chronic mental illness or substance use is in the home. Reunification in cases of abuse and neglect often creates significant ethical dilemmas for APNs. Two competing narratives forwarded by foster parents stand out: The first was the case of a small child, a 2 1/2-year-old girl who slipped her soft hand in mine when it was time to eat lunch during one of my parenting classes. It was relayed that her mother had almost killed her, and she had been hospitalized "for a long time." The court still had not decided whether the child would return to her mother. The second story was of an incarcerated woman who had just given birth and had a substance use disorder. She paid her debt to society while the foster parents cared for her infant. On her release from prison, the mother secured employment, cared for her child, and remained "clean" from substances. The foster parents helped her by babysitting whenever she needed them to and offered emotional support. The two families became friends and partners. These very different situations speak to the human elements of how to determine what is in the best interest of the child.

In reunions in which adult adopted individuals seek to find birth relatives, options include social media and Internet reunion registries (see the Introduction). Stories of such reunions also reflect visual recordings and documentaries. A whole genre of YouTube videos and other documentaries (about reunions and adoption in general) is available. Adopted persons are finding their voices through these communication modes to tell their stories of growing up in adopted households and to record their journeys of reunion with birth family members.

CASE STUDIES: THE CHILD/ADULT WHO IS ADOPTED

□ □ □ □

CASE STUDY 1: AMANUEL

In Ethiopia, birthdates are not usually celebrated and births and deaths may not be recorded. Amanuel's adoptive parents were told that he was 2 years old; however, after being home for 6 months, his parents have noticed that his gross motor development seems to be of an older child. The medical records are unclear, and it is not certain what his birth weight was. Malnourishment was a known problem before his grandmother, old and ill herself, brought Amanuel to the local orphanage for care. She turned in the papers of relinquishment from his dying mother, stating that the father had died from AIDS last month. In the orphanage, he was taken under the care of a U.S. adoption agency and subsequently had a medical exam that revealed malnutrition and a negative ELISA HIV test.

Amanuel officially stepped on U.S. soil on April 10. On arrival, the medical exam revealed lice and intestinal parasites, and it was noted that his uvula had been removed, a fairly common practice in Ethiopia. Amanuel's adoptive parents treated the infectious diseases (lice and Giardia) and monitored his weight and growth patterns closely. The adoption medicine specialist confirmed his immunization status either through antibody titers or revaccinations for diphtheria, tetanus, polio, hepatitis B, chicken pox, measles, mumps, and rubella. An HIV ELISA with reflex Western Blot and a qualitative PCR HIV DNA was also ordered. These results were negative.

Months passed, and Amanuel transitioned from Amharic to English fairly easily; his adoptive parents had learned a few words in his native language, which helped him feel less isolated. However, his mother, Lucy, found that Amanuel would not let her console him when he gets hurt, and he regresses when there is any change in his routine. For example, when the parents decided to change to a different day care, Amanuel threw tantrums, kicking, screaming, and trying to bite his mother as she tried to take him into the new building. He refuses to sit at the dinner table at times and throws his toys when he is reprimanded for not obeying his parents.

As the first-year anniversary of his arrival home approaches, his parents note that his affect is sad and he seems withdrawn. He often colors, but has difficulty holding the crayons at times. Lucy notices there are two outlines of larger figures in most of his drawings. When questioned who they might be, Amanuel shakes his head and leaves the room. Recently, Amanuel has been cooking dinner and baking cookies with his mother, an activity that he greatly enjoys.

Lucy brings him for his 3-year well child examination to his pediatric nurse practitioner, Adele. The toddler refuses to hold his mother's hand, and she gently has hold of his arm to ensure his safety.

APN Next Steps

Adele notes Amanuel's height and weight show a positive curve on the growth chart, and he appears well nourished and hydrated. However, because of his history of malnourishment, she decides to check blood values to rule out anemia. He is due for the hepatitis B and pneumococcal conjugate vaccinations as well. She attempts to perform the physical examination; however, Amanuel refuses to allow her to touch him and screams when she attempts to palpate for lymph node enlargement in the neck area as part of his routine examination. Adele decides to withdraw from the examination and take a more detailed history of Amanuel's behaviors.

His mother reports increasing resistance to instructions and sleep disturbances. "He is also really distracted. Even a bit hyperactive at times. And he was never a cuddly child, but he really doesn't like to be touched. In fact, he wants nothing to touch his skin—he loves being naked!"

Adele understands these symptoms could be attributed to a number of potential diagnoses, even autistism spectrum disorder, sensory processing disorder, or pediatric depression and posttraumatic stress disorder (PTSD). She understands the little boy has been exposed to several ACEs. A limited physical exam is eventually completed because of Amanuel's resistance and to avoid further emotional trauma. A Denver II Developmental Screening Test is also performed (Frankenburg, Dodds, Archer, Shapiro, & Bresnick, 1992); several deficits and delays are noted, including an inability to build a tower of eight cubes, and to put on his shirt independently. Adele also knows that these instructions may be negatively influenced by Amanuel's receptive language. A referral is made to a developmental-behavioral pediatrician to assess for the potential diagnoses already mentioned and to determine whether an occupational therapy evaluation for sensory issues is warranted. Lucy is also encouraged to consider behavioral counseling once the referral evaluations are obtained. Lastly, Adele coaches Lucy that Amanuel is nearing the 1-year anniversary of his arrival home. Some children become withdrawn and appear sad as this anniversary draws near. Adele encourages continued activities such as cooking together and to use these times as opportunities to have Amanuel describe how he used to spend time with his family in Ethiopia, taking cues from the little boy as to what he wants to talk about. Adele, as an adoption-informed caregiver, knows that building on the strengths between the mother and son will help to foster Amanuel's feelings of competency, safety, and connection.

□ □ □ □

CASE STUDY 2: CHRISTI

Christi, 12 years old, does not have many friends and is bullied at her middle school for being overweight. She is attention seeking and has been diagnosed with attention deficit hyperactivity disorder (ADHD) and depression. She is stable on atomoxetine HCl at 60 mg daily and is being assessed regularly for signs of suicidal ideation. Christi has been seen on a regular basis by the psychiatric mental health nurse practitioner, Helen. Although she has been with her adoptive parents since the age of 6, Christi has been increasingly oppositional and defiant, lying to her parents about where she is and what she is doing. Her grades have dropped recently to Cs and Ds. Never a child who liked to be hugged or touched, she now rejects any physical affection from her parents.

Recently, her adoptive mother found marijuana in her room and a note to her "birth mother" wondering why she was "given up." Although there has been an open adoption agreement between her adoptive parents and her birth mother, Christi has not seen or heard from her birth mother in 4 years. Records have documented the abuse (beatings) and neglect (food insecurity) that led to her removal from the home, but Christi denies remembering much of the trauma. She has a half-sibling in another state that she does not want any contact with. As a young adolescent, Christi is constantly on alert for signs of danger, a steady state that has exhausted her. She has difficulty trusting others, which has led to peer relationship discord, and she reports nightmares of events that she cannot describe or accurately recall.

Her adoptive mother and father have grown increasingly concerned, but feel helpless. Helen, an adoption-competent and trauma-informed practitioner, understands how the past and present trauma (bullying) are potentially affecting Christi's acting-out behaviors.

APN Next Steps

First, Helen performs a psychiatric evaluation, including a focus on signs of suicidal ideation or plans: "Have you ever wished you weren't alive anymore?" and progressing to asking of any thoughts of self-harm or violence toward others. The answers are negative. With the family's permission, she speaks to school personnel and Christi's pediatric nurse practitioner, gathering collateral information. She also speaks with each family member individually, including Christi. She rules out a psychiatric comorbidity and learns that Christi has been very confused since her biological mother made contact with her, which she did not share with her adoptive family.

She then begins to educate both Christi and her parents on how the trauma Christi experienced as a young child is affecting her life. The APN provides an overview of trauma-informed care, understanding that abuse and neglect affect the brain's neurodevelopment and, therefore, patterns of behavior. Helen realizes that a therapist trained in trauma-informed treatment with experience working with adoptive families is needed to work with this family. She refers Christi for individual counseling by a trauma-informed therapist to address her depressive symptoms as well as a substance use evaluation. She also refers Christi's family to an experienced therapist in helping them recover from trauma.

Over the course of several months as Christi is seen for medication evaluation visits, Helen encourages her to express her feelings and evaluates her progress in therapy. Helen assesses Christi's mood dysphoria for symptoms of PTSD, major depressive disorder, generalized anxiety disorder, and panic disorder. Her substance use evaluation revealed one-time use and did not recommend outpatient treatment at this time, but did recommend close follow-up. Helen diagnoses Christi with PTSD and begins a low-dose selective serotonin reuptake inhibitor (SSRI). Most recently, Christi reports "feeling better" with a more appropriate affect. Her parents' feedback confirms this; they also describe Christi as more compliant at home and involved in more family activities. Together, they have reached out to Christi's birth mother. Christi's parents understand how important this is to her, and, with close communications between them, have allowed her to take the lead on this contact.

□ □ □ □

CASE STUDY 3: WILLIAM

William does not remember much about his early childhood—at least the 12 months he spent in foster care before being adopted by Ben and Maddy, a White couple who struggled with infertility. William's upbringing was a happy one filled with time spent at the family's lakeside cabin and fishing with his father. Both Ben and Maddy are teachers at the local community college and have a large extended family. They did not see any problem with a transracial adoption (William is Black). Despite protests from his parents, some family members did not recognize William's place as equal to other grandchildren within the family. Still, that was the only type of "difference" he was exposed to in his childhood.

As a 20-year-old man majoring in mechanical engineering, he presents at his university's health care clinic for complaints of severe muscle pain after working out. College has been difficult for him as he has struggled to understand racial undertones from peers and outright hostility from strangers. The university lacks diversity, but he did not expect the uneven reception he had received 2 years ago as a freshman. His parents smoothed it over by emphasizing that he is there to get an education and not to worry about what others think. Still, he is feeling a new alienation from them, an emotional distance, as he makes decisions about whom to date and what friends he is most comfortable with.

Since coming to college, he began to run a few miles every night. It helped with the stress of the coursework and the solitude allowed him to think. But once he arrived back at his apartment, he experienced pains in his legs almost every night after running.

The primary care pediatric nurse practitioner, Mallory, at the student health center completes William's physical assessment, and aside from these symptoms, his assessment is within normal limits. However, she knows his symptoms need to be further evaluated. In addition to a full lab panel, Mallory orders a blood test to confirm William's sickle cell trait, which he recorded in his health history. Mallory knows that each state has guidelines for newborn screening tests, but when she asks William if he is aware of previous screenings, he responds that he is unaware of any. Although sickle cell is routinely screened for today in William's state of residence, Mallory is unsure whether William was previously screened as an infant. William informs her that his medical file while in foster care was missing several important documents, including some of his newborn information. A routine blood test at the time of his adoption found the sickle cell trait, and his parents ensured that he knew about this genetic trait.

APN Next Steps

Mallory's confirmation is received when William's test comes back positive for sickle cell trait. She reviews ways to minimize these symptoms with him—drinking plenty of fluids, stopping exercising if pain or breathlessness begins, and if he adds exercises to his workout, doing so gradually. She then reviews what sickle cell trait is: He received one sickle cell gene from one of his birth parents. He does not have sickle cell anemia and will not develop the disease, but he should use this information if he decides to start a family of his own. If his partner also carries this trait, their children will be at 50% risk for carrying the trait and 25% risk for sickle cell disease.

William seems distraught, and Mallory senses there is more to his unease than just this news. He confides in her that he has been considering a full-blown "genetic workup" ever since coming to college and heard of direct-to-consumer companies that will do genetic tests through the mail.

He states, "It is like this identity thing right now. I mean, I was raised White, but sure don't look like it. Sometimes, I don't really know what I am. Now, I find out that my health is impacted by this genetic trait, and I wonder what else is in my DNA."

Mallory is aware that as an adopted person, there are dimensions to William's care that surpass the physical and extend into issues of culture, race, identity, and self-concept. First Mallory asks for additional background information, for example, whether William's parents discussed issues of race and class with him as he grew up. Often, transracial adoptions require purposeful cross-cultural interactions and preparedness for when an adopted person enters into society in an independent way. The safety net of the middle-class neighborhood where William grew up has been left behind, and he is experiencing his identity in reflections of others with whom he is unfamiliar. Interpreting these reactions will require William to continue a dialogue with his parents, his peers, and others in society. Ultimately, he will need to create a path that is most comfortable for him.

Mallory is able to refer William to a health care genetic counselor who practices in the community. The counselor can advise the best approach for further genetic testing, including proprietary companies. She is also able to offer William literature and books that have been written specifically for transracially adopted individuals and their families, such as *In Their Own Voices: Transracial Adoptees Tell Their Stories* (2000) and *In Their Voices: Black Americans on Transracial Adoption* (2015) by Rhonda Roorda. Mallory schedules a follow-up with William in 2 weeks to assess his muscular pain; she also refers him to the student services counselor so that he can continue his journey toward self-identity with support. Last, she ensures that he is aware of the cultural center on campus that might be able to connect him with resources as he explores his racial identity and navigates society away from the protective layer of his parents.

□ □ □ □

CASE STUDY 4: JACOB

Jacob is 28 years old and enjoys his career as a very successful medical device sales person. He had always known he was adopted and did not feel particularly close to his adoptive parents, who live out of state. He sends them cards on holidays and tries to get home around Christmas. He was adopted as an infant and matched to parents whose background was compatible with his birth mother's values—at least that is what he has been told. The adoption was facilitated by an attorney who was a professional acquaintance of his father, also an attorney. When he was 18 years old, his adoptive mother shared his birth parents' information with Jacob, stating that they had both indicated agreement to being located if that was what Jacob wanted. He never pursued finding his birth parents.

College was a fun time during which he joined a social fraternity while earning As and Bs in his business school coursework. Sales fit him well as rejection did not seem to affect him or his ego. People's impressions of him were usually based on his handsome features and fit body. He believes he has earned the right to look good in a suit because he works out on a daily basis. Socially, he has never wanted for friends, but could not really identify a "best bud." He recently broke off a 2-year engagement with a woman whom he said was getting too "clingy." Since then, he has engaged in fairly frequent, unprotected sex and comes to see his adult/gerontology primary nurse practitioner for complaints of burning on urination.

APN Next Steps

The A-GNP, Sonia, first listens closely to Jacob's presenting problems. She notes that he seems nonchalant about his symptoms, and she continues to ask about the onset, duration, intensity, and frequency of his symptoms. She then uses the Brief Sexual History Tool (Lanier et al., 2014) to take a complete history and to collect additional information. She then conducts a focused history of presenting symptoms and a physical assessment, examining his genitals for outward legions or blisters. After listening to Jacob's symptoms, particularly his urethritis, she decides to collect a urine specimen and order a nucleic acid amplification test (NAAT) for both *Chlamydia trachomatis* and *Neisseria gonorrhoeae*, plus a syphilis and an HIV screen.

Jacob's demeanor radically changes as he is horrified that he may have a sexually transmitted infection (STI) or an HIV infection. He becomes agitated, saying, "Oh, my God. What have I done?" Sonia listens to Jacob's distress, providing a calm demeanor.

He begins to speak rapidly, "I just cannot believe this. What if the tests are positive? What if I have some incurable disease?"

Sonia matter-of-factly and gently educates Jacob on each test, answering his questions, which include the treatment/management if the test(s) are positive. She also instructs Jacob on safe sex practices and that if he is HIV positive, but not yet at a level detectable with a test, he could pass the infection onto partners. She emphasizes how important safe sex practices are and explains those to him. He nods and says, "Okay. Yes. I understand."

When the test results arrive, Sonia calls Jacob to communicate that he is positive for chlamydia and will order azithromycin, 1 gram single dose. She would like to see him in 3 months for a follow-up HIV test to rule out a window period of recent infection.

He again becomes agitated, "I have to wait 3 months to see if I'm HIV positive?" Sonia explains that if he is recently infected, the test may not accurately reflect his health status.

Follow-Up

Jacob returns to see Sonia and receive his HIV test results, which are negative. He exhales a long breath as he is told, but adds, "I've been buying those drugstore kits and they've been negative."

Sonia notes a change in Jacob. He looks fatigued and a bit disheveled, but also presents in a more authentic way—the bravado is gone. "I've kind of been examining my life. Did you know I was adopted?"

Sonia was not aware. Jacob had been given complete medical records from his birth mother that disclosed his maternal and paternal families' medical histories and thus had been able to complete his health history. He tells her he has been reading "like crazy" about how adoption can influence a person, especially attachment to others and intimate relationships.

He states, "I kind of feel like I've been running all my life. I'm not sure from what."

The test results and the possibility of having a serious medical condition prompted Jacob to reflect on why he could not establish close relationships with others, something his ex-girlfriend had accused him of.

Sonia, who is an adoption-competent provider, reflects on what Jacob is telling her. She summarizes and adds, "I know this has been a difficult time for you. But you've taken this potential health care crisis and worked hard to understand your behaviors and interpersonal patterns. I hope you feel good about this. It took a lot of courage for you to do this." She goes on to describe how adopted persons make sense of their lives in different ways. Some bury their adoption histories inside whereas others are able to openly process it. And some, such as Jacob, are unaware for a long time of the issues that need to be addressed.

He also called his adoptive mother so that she could again share his birth parents' contact information. In the past 3 months, he had located his mother; his father passed away 2 years ago. He had flown to Florida to see his birth mother, who was ecstatic to meet her adult son. He is also making an effort to connect emotionally with his adoptive parents and reconnect with his ex-girlfriend. Last, he is seeing a therapist who understands the dynamics of adult adoptions and is making progress on his identity and "forging bonds with others."

APNS' CARE OF THE CHILD/ADULT WHO IS ADOPTED

As this chapter has described, physical, psychological, social, and spiritual needs unique to being an adopted person exist and have implications for the delivery of care by APNs. Adopted persons are heterogeneous and have encountered a wide variety of experiences before coming to live with their adoptive parents, which may include transracial placements, trauma, maltreatment, and multiple caregivers. Often marginalized, adopted individuals should be given a voice, options, and control whenever possible (Table 5.1).

TABLE 5.1   *Child/Adult Who Is Adopted: What to Look for and What to Do*

The Child/Adult Who Is Adopted
What to Look For (Assessment):
☐ Follow assessment guidelines as outlined in Chapter 2 and per the American Academy of Pediatrics.
☐ Assess adverse childhood experiences (ACE) indicators in adopted children and adults whose history indicates the potential for trauma.
☐ Monitor for signs of psychological distress, including depression, suicidal ideation/plans, and substance use disorders.
☐ Tease out physical complaints that may be related to psychosocial needs.
☐ Assess for microaggressions against transracial adopted individuals and those with sexual minority parents.
What to Do (Management):
☐ Provide psychosocial support and therapeutic communication before and after placement.
☐ Support reunion and reunification efforts as appropriate.
☐ Encourage adopted persons to have a voice in placement and afterward.
☐ Practice with an understanding that adoption is a transformative, lifelong process.
☐ Refer adoptive children, adolescents, and adults to needed resources to strengthen their role in society.
☐ Provide continuity of services for patients who are adopted individuals through patient-centered medical homes.

CHAPTER HIGHLIGHTS

☐ Demographically, adopted children are more likely to be from racial minorities than the general population. They are also more likely to live in households with parents who have higher incomes and more education.

☐ Two current trends in access for adopted persons are unsealing birth certificates and open adoption arrangements.

☐ Genetic testing before adoption is controversial, with proponents on each side asserting ethical implications: best interest of the child and preparedness of the adoptive parents.

☐ Adopted persons are increasingly seeking out genetic testing.

☐ Adopted persons may have parents of different race/ethnic groups as well as sexual minority parents.

☐ Psychological issues in adopted children, adolescents, and adults have been studied for many decades. A disproportionate number of behavior issues have been identified; however, the reasons for these issues are not entirely clear.

☐ Trauma experiences and adverse childhood experiences are key factors in the development and health of adopted individuals.

☐ Adopted children's and adolescent's ability to answer questions competently empowers them. One tool is the W.I.S.E Up! Tool.

☐ Increasingly, reunions are occurring between birth parents and adopted individuals.

Questions for Reflection

Following are a few questions to reflect upon. You can use these to start a journal for yourself or in a classroom discussion with peers and the instructor.

1. As a society, how do we address the trauma and the aftermath of ACEs? How can APNs work to reverse the increasing evidence of trauma in our country?

2. What are your beliefs and feelings about genetic testing for individuals who are being considered for adoption? On what basis do you support such beliefs? Are they similar to what would be screened for in nonadopted persons? How could you defend your position with colleagues and patients?

3. How do you define psychological issues within the context of adoption?
4. What factors should be weighed in matching children with adoptive parents? What constitutes in the "best interest of the child"?
5. How can nurses empower children and adolescents when they are faced with obtrusive, and even rude, questions about their past?
6. What case study spoke to you the most? Why? What personal and professional feelings were evoked within you?

References

23andMe. (2016). We bring the world of genetics to you. Retrieved from www.23andme.com

325Kamra, Inc. (2016). Reuniting families through DNA. Retrieved from www.325kamra.org/about

Allen, D. W., Pakaluk, C., & Price, J. (2013). Nontraditional families and childhood progress through school: A comment on Rosenfeld. *Demography, 50,* 955–961. doi:10.1007/s13524-012-0169-x

American Nurses Association & The International Society of Nurses in Genetics. (2016). *Genetics/genomics nursing: Scope and standards of practice* (2nd ed.). Silver Spring, MD: Author.

American Society of Human Genetics Social Issues Committee & The American College of Medical Genetics Social, Ethical, and Legal Issues Committee. (2000). ASHG/ACMG statement: Genetic testing in adoption. *American Journal of Human Genetics, 66,* 761–767.

Baden, A. L., & O'Leary Wiley, M. (2007). Counseling adopted persons in adulthood: Integrating practice and research. *The Counseling Psychologist, 35*(6), 868–901. doi: 10.1177/0011000006291409

Bramlett, M. D., Radel, L. F., & Blumberg, S. J. (2007). The health and well-being of adopted children. *Pediatrics, 119,* S54–S60.

Brodinsky, D. (2015). *The modern adoptive families study.* New York, NY: The Donaldson Adoption Institute. Retrieved from adoptioninstitute.org /wordpress/wp-content/uploads/2015/09/DAI_MAF_Report_090115_ R7_Edit.pdf

Center for Adoption Support and Education. (n.d). *WISE Up!* Retrieved from http://adoptionsupport.org/education-resources/for-professionals/c-s-e -publications/w-i-s-e-up

Centers for Disease Control and Prevention. (2016). About the CDC-Kaiser ACE study. Retrieved from www.cdc.gov/violenceprevention/acestudy /about.html

Child Welfare Information Gateway. (2016). Foster care statistics 2014. Retrieved from www.childwelfare.gov/pubs/factsheets/foster

Donaldson Adoption Institute. (2016). Open letter: Adoption. Retrieved from www.letsadoptreform.org/open-letter

Ela, E. J. (2011). *Adoptive parents in the U.S., 2007* (FP-11-05). National Center for Family and Marriage Research. Retrieved from ncfmr.bgsu.edu /pdf/family_profiles/file 99071.pdf.

Farr, R. H., Crain, E. E., Oakley, M. K., Cashen, K. K., & Garber, K. J. (2016). Microaggressions, feelings of difference, and resilience among adopted children with sexual minority parents. *Journal of Youth and Adolescence, 45*, 85–104. doi:10.1007/s10964-015-0353-6

Farr, R. H., & Patterson, C. J. (2009). Transracial adoption by lesbian, gay, and heterosexual couples: Who completes transracial adoptions and with what results? *Adoption Quarterly, 12*, 187–204. doi:10.1080/10926750903313328

Felitti, V. J., Anda, R. F., Nordenberg, D., Williamson, D. F., Spitz, A. M., Edwards, V., . . . Marks, J. S. (1998). Relationship of childhood abuse and household dysfunction to many of the leading causes of death in adults: The Adverse Childhood Experiences (ACE) study. *American Journal of Preventive Medicine, 14*(4), 245–258.

Forster, A. K., Foli, K. J., Abrahamson, K., & Richards, E. (2016). Brief report: Adults who are adopted: Implications for nurse practitioners. *Journal for Nurse Practitioners, 12*, e351–e353.

Fox, B. H., Perez, N., Cass, E., Baglivio, M. T., & Epps, N. (2015). Trauma changes everything: Examining the relationship between childhood experiences and serious, violent and chronic juvenile offenders. *Child Abuse & Neglect, 46*, 163–173. doi:10.1016/j.chiabu.2015.01.011

Frankenburg, W. K., Dodds, J., Archer, P., Shapiro, H., & Bresnick, B. (1992). The DENVER II: A major revision and restandardization of the Denver Developmental Screening Test. *Pediatrics, 89*(1):91–97.

Lanier, Y., Castellanos, T., Barrow, R. Y., Jordan, W. C., Caine, V., & Sutton, M. Y. (2014). Brief sexual histories and routine HIV/STD testing by medical providers. *Aids Patient Care and STDs, 28*(3), 113–120. doi:10.1089/apc.2013.0328

Maternal-Child-Health Inter Divisional Council of Colorado League for Nursing. (1961). *The role of the nurse in relinquishments and adoptions in Colorado: 1961*. Wheat Ridge, CO: Colorado League for Nursing.

McGuinness, T.M., & Dyer, J.G. (2006). International adoption as a natural experiment. *Journal of Pediatric Nursing, 21*(4), 276–288. doi:10.1016/j.pedn.2006.02.001

McGuinness, T.M., McGuinness, J.P., & Dyer, J.G. (2000). Risk and protective factors in children adopted from the former Soviet Union. *Journal of Pediatric Health Care, 14*(3), 109–116. doi:10.1067/mph.2000.103291

McGuinness, T.M., & Pallansch, L. (2007). Problem behaviors of children adopted from the former Soviet Union. *Journal of Pediatric Health Care, 21*(3), 171–179. doi:10.1016/j.pedhc.2006.05.008

McGuinness, T.M., & Robinson, C.B. (2011). Update on international adoption: Focus on Russia. *Journal of Psychosocial Nursing and Mental Health Services, 49*(6), 17–20. doi:10.3928/02793695-20110503-02

Prickett, K. C., Martin-Storey, A., & Crosnoe, R. (2015). A research note on time with children in different- and same-sex two-parent families. *Demography, 52*, 905–918. doi:10.1007/s13524-015-0385-2

Roorda, R. (2000). *In their own voices: Transracial adoptees tell their stories.* New York, NY: Columbia University Press.

Roorda, R. (2015). *In their voices: Black Americans on transracial adoption.* New York, NY: Columbia University Press.

Rosenfeld, M. J. (2010). Nontraditional families and childhood progress through school. *Demography, 47*(3), 755–775.

Schoettle, M. (2000). *W.I.S.E. Up! powerbook.* Burtonsville, MD: Center for Adoption Support and Education.

Singer, E. (2010). The "W.I.S.E. Up" tool: Empowering children to cope with questions and comments about adoption. *Pediatric Nursing, 36*(4), 209–212.

Taylor, P. G. (2008). Pre-adoptive genetic testing: Is the current policy too restrictive? *Families in Society: The Journal of Contemporary Social Sciences, 89*(3), 360–365. doi:10.1606/1044-3894.3761

Vandivere, S., Malm, K., & Radel, L. (2009). *Adoption USA: A chartbook based on the 2007 National Survey of Adoptive Parents.* Washington, DC: The U.S. Department of Health and Human Services, Office of the Assistant Secretary for Planning and Evaluation.

6

Kinship Parents

□ □ □ □

PURPOSE OF THE CHAPTER

In this chapter, we explore the role and needs of kinship parents, a unique, vulnerable, diverse population with health risk factors compounded by the responsibilities of raising children as older adults. Kinship caregiving is somewhat new to our lexicon, but such parenting is not new in practice. Think of the novel *The Wizard of Oz* (Baum, 1900), in which Dorothy is parented by Aunt Em and Uncle Henry. There appears to be an emotional arc to the connection between Aunt Em and Dorothy as their relationship becomes closer, and ultimately ends with Dorothy wanting to return home to her kinship caregivers, not unlike the kinship relationships we see today.

This chapter introduces four individuals in case studies who have assumed the role of the parent. They span a spectrum of legal arrangements based on the birth parents' presence in the home and in the family. Each has diverse backgrounds that include various challenges related to being a kinship parent: a 68-year-old grandmother who is recovering from orthopedic surgery; an older, middle-aged man who is caring for his grandchildren while his daughter is on military deployment; a 61-year-old woman who has assumed the care of her stepgrandchildren; and an older adult who is victim to elder abuse at the hands of her kinship children. Cases are described, followed by the identified issues and concerns that are amenable to nursing interventions.

Learning Objectives

At the completion of the chapter, the reader will be able to:

1. Discuss comparisons of demographic factors between kinship parents and general households with at least one parent
2. Compare and contrast the family dynamics of kinship foster care with nonrelative foster care
3. Identify kinship family risk factors that are amenable to advanced practice nurse (APN) management or referral, such as food insecurity
4. Be familiar with caregiver burden, depression, stress, and the health effects for older adults/kinship caregivers
5. Describe the assessment and mandatory actions when elder abuse is suspected/discovered

OVERVIEW OF KINSHIP PARENTS

As a profession, nurses are increasingly called upon to contribute to a culture of health, prevent disease, and promote well-being. Although these are worthy goals, nurses have to address the basic needs of individuals and families first (think Maslow's Hierarchy of Needs). You cannot consider self-actualization if you do not have enough air to breath, or enough food to eat. The reality of widespread food insecurity in the United States is startling, with 19.2% of households with children experiencing food insecurity (U.S. Department of Agriculture: Economic Research Service, 2015). As the level of poverty increases, so does the percentage of households that face food insecurity, up to 33.7% (U.S. Department of Agriculture: Economic Research Service, 2015). Many of these are households maintained by kinship parents. In fact, 24% of children are adopted by relatives (Vandivere et al., 2009).

In 2014, foster care provided by a relative jumped to 29% of all foster care placements in the United States (Child Welfare Information Gateway, 2016). This figure does not include kinship parents who are not officially accessing the foster care/child welfare system. Kinship parents represent a vulnerable and quickly growing population, which has seen an 18% increase in the last decade (Annie E. Casey Foundation, 2012). It is also fairly common in society: 9% of children will live with extended family for at least 3 consecutive months before they turn 18 years of age (Annie E. Casey Foundation, 2012). Economically, these families are disadvantaged. Compared with children living with at least one parent, kinship families are more likely to live below the poverty line (22% and 38%, respectively). But the statistics become even more worrisome when extreme poverty is considered: 43% of children with at least one parent versus 63% of kinship households live below the 200% poverty line. The Annie E. Casey Foundation (2012) reports that: "According to U.S. Census Bureau data, kinship caregivers are more likely to be poor, single, older, less educated, and unemployed than families in which at least one parent is present" (p. 4). In addition, many of these children have experienced trauma and adverse childhood experiences (ACEs). This creates a dynamic picture of the potential for multiple patients within one family unit.

Kinship caregivers, who are often grandparents, feel an acute stigma. As director of a project that delivered trauma-informed parenting classes to kinship parents in rural Indiana counties, I heard narratives, reflections of pain and shame at the events that necessitated the removal of children from their birth parents who were often, the kinship parents' own children. Drug use, death, incarceration, and immaturity were often cited as reasons why these grandparents were now raising their grandchildren. Blurred lines of who are "mom" and "dad," and new labels of how to refer to the kinship caregivers are agreed upon within the families. Generations learn new boundaries, young aunts and uncles are now siblings, and power is redistributed and negotiated. Legal issues are considered, and often reconsidered. In some of the parenting classes, nonrelative foster parents sat alongside kinship parents. The differences were significant. Boundaries of the families themselves and the multigenerational dynamics present within the family system differed between relative and nonrelative foster care families. The nonrelative foster parents rendered care, knowing the child's placement was probably temporary, and during this time, their role was to provide a safe, nurturing environment while the child's birth parents could not. (Table 6.1 presents the differences between kinship care and traditional foster care.) Kinship parents spoke of feeling uncertainty about whether the arrangement would be permanent or temporary, the drain on their finances, being less knowledgeable about services, and ill-prepared to parent children with significant behavioral issues.

TABLE 6.1 *Kinship Care Versus Traditional Foster Care*

KINSHIP CARE	TRADITIONAL FOSTER CARE
Prexisting relationship with child	No preexisting relationship with child
Redefines existing family relationships	Strengthens new family relationships
Mixed feelings about loss of parent to child	Celebration of a new family
Mixed feelings about loss of role as grandparent, aunt, uncle, etc.	Excitement about new role as parent
Knowledge of family dynamics	Limited knowledge of family dynamics
Decision to become a caregiver is unplanned and in crisis; request from parent, child protection or courts	Decision to become a caregiver is planned and voluntary
Limited preparation for caregiving	Preparation for caregiving role and support already in place before child is placed in home
Unanticipated requirements to become a foster or adoptive parent	Requirements to become foster or adoptive parent are anticipated
Guilt over birth parent problems	No guilt over birth parent problems
Guilt for taking over parental role for the child	Feelings that they are saving the child
Perception that they are betraying the birth parent by assuming legal relationships	Feeling they are displaying loyalty and commitment to the child by assuming legal relationship
In competition with birth parent if the child becomes attached to relative	Motivated to demonstrate attachment that is as strong as previous attachment with birth parent
Split loyalties and hesitation to legalize relationship	High motivation to legalize relationship

Source: ChildFocus® and The North American Council on Adoptable Children (2010).

During one of the modules in the parenting class, we discuss compassion fatigue that kinship parents may experience through their empathy toward the children under their care who have been abused and neglected. Sadness, shame, frustration, anger, exhaustion, and fear are among the emotions elicited when caregivers' empathize on a continual, relentless basis. After having the parents discuss what they listed in response to caring for their children, one parent commented: "I don't see one listed here that's important: guilt." She was right. For kinship parents, there is often pronounced guilt from perceived mistakes when parenting the birth parents and an attribution of the current situation to these mistakes.

Resources and support are sometimes scarce, and informal networks may be created as a result. I had asked the class participants where I might be able to distribute information about the classes, because recruitment had been a challenge. I wanted to reach folks who might benefit from the information. One quickly said, "Go to the McDonald's. There's a bunch of us there. They have that big indoor playground. You should see all us kinship folks with our kids. They just play and play." Another volunteer in one rural community had advised me to be sure to distribute the fliers at food pantries around the area.

There are also safety issues, which can take various forms. First, kinship parents report being a buffer, a gatekeeper, and a protector of the children whose care they have assumed from the birth parents who no longer can or will care for them. This is especially important if the parent has a substance use disorder. One kinship parent that I spoke with emphasized that only supervised parental visits were allowed with his two grandchildren. And such visits were no longer occurring in his home. He drove the children to a public space for their safety, as he believed behaviors were often better in public places. Second, the behaviors of the child may place the older kinship parent at risk. Evidence of hitting, biting, punching, and bruising should be thoroughly investigated if assessed upon evaluation by the APN—for the both child and the adult. The children who display aggressive behaviors may be mimicking in play what they have witnessed or experienced in their homes and need to be referred to a mental health professional for evaluation and services.

Additionally, the safety of the child has to be considered with kinship placement. When speaking to a group of youth workers in a rural county, staff from the Department of Child Services (DCS) described how they make every effort to find relatives and strongly desire relative placements. Yet, they added, there were occasions when the kinship parents could not pass a criminal background check. Awareness of and prioritizing safety for both the kinship provider and the child are critical for APNs when evaluating patients, both old and young, who are in kinship arrangements.

TYPOLOGIES OF KINSHIP FAMILIES

There appear to be patterns or typologies of kinship families. Using foster family data from the State of Illinois, Zinn (2010) revealed four classes of kinship parents or typologies employing latent class statistical analysis. The first class, "empty nest grandparents," the largest group at 41%, is comprised of grandparents or great-grandparents who are more often married with very few non–foster children in the home. These individuals are most likely to experience health problems. The second class, "parenting grandparents," families are also headed by great- or grandparents and contain at least one non–foster care child. Compared with the other classes, the presence of additional adults in the home is high. The third class, "collateral kin with some children" families, are less likely to be headed by partnered adults, but there are other adults in the home. The reverse was found for the fourth class, or "parenting collateral kin," families: They are less likely to be headed by partnered adults and have no other adults in the home (p. 331). Two important variables that were statistically significant in supplementary analysis were relatedness of family members and the number of nonfoster care children in the homes; these two items may help further define kinship family typologies (Zinn, 2010). APNs may find such categories helpful when evaluating older adult kinship parents and their social support.

CAREGIVING GRANDMOTHERS

Grandparents experience a spectrum of emotions and stress in their role as kinship parents. The work of Carol Musil and colleagues should be noted. Another notable nurse leader in this area is Susan Kelley, whose work with African American grandmothers provides evidence to support APN practice. The journal *GrandFamilies: The Contemporary Journal of Research, Practice and Policy* is a source of information for APNs as they provide care to this unique group of individuals. These contributions to nursing science and practice have significantly increased our understanding of caregiving grandmothers' overall experiences, caregiver burden, and interventions to support optimal health. Caregiving grandmothers reported stress and depression as emotional health outcomes (Musil et al., 2010; Musil, Warner, Zauszniewski, Wykle, &

Standing, 2009). The burden of caregiving is significant, especially over time: Grandmothers who assumed primary care of a grandchild experienced the most stress, intrafamily strain, and perceived problems in family functioning; worsening health and increased stress were also revealed over a 24-month period (Musil et al., 2010). However, depressive symptoms and interfamily strains were found to be mediated by resourcefulness in caregiving grandmothers who were studied over a 5-year period (Musil, Jeanblanc, Burant, Zauszniewski, & Warner, 2013). Resourcefulness training (RT) of caregiving grandmothers using both written and verbal disclosure (tape recordings) was overall effective in reducing perceived stress, depressive symptoms, and enhancing quality of life (Zauszniewski, Musil, Burant, & Au, 2014). A pilot study of an online RT revealed overall positive results; however, modifications, such as support for participants when the study is initiated, were recommended (Musil, Zauszniewski, Burant, Toly, & Warner, 2015). More research is needed to continue to test what appears to be a promising intervention, RT, to support caregiving grandmothers.

REASONS WHY KINSHIP CARE EXISTS

For many kinship parents, parenting responsibilities are taken on suddenly and unexpectedly. For others, there is knowledge that families are unstable and in crisis. The DCS is charged with seeking out relatives in order to place children who have been removed from the home. Relatives are then left with the dilemma of caring for the child or placing them in the child welfare system with nonfamily caregivers. From those kinship parents whom I have interacted with, the latter option is often unpalatable: "I didn't want a stranger raising him. I couldn't stand that thought." Yet the children can present with significant histories of maltreatment with thoughts, emotions, and behaviors that sometimes transform the lives of the kinship provider. For example, grandparents have expressed that their friends and other extended family members rejected them, either because of loyalty to the birth parents or because of the child's behaviors at social events. The grandparents were left feeling their support systems had been taken from them when they needed their friends and family the most. One grandmother said, "I was so hurt when our friends didn't want to socialize with us anymore. My husband

and I used to be so social. I don't know that I'm over it and they left us years ago. At the same time, I don't know that I'd ever want them in my life again."

As previously discussed, family structures vary: Kinship care may be informal and temporary or ultimately result in permanent placement. Whatever the arrangement, we do know children have better outcomes overall when placed with kinship care than with nonrelative foster care arrangements. There are strengths to care provided by kin: Children progressed better with behavioral and social skills problems (Sakai, Lin, & Flores, 2011). Kinship care offers children the benefits of familiar caregivers, continuity of family and cultural traditions, decreased trauma from separation, reinforced identity and self-esteem, reduction of racial disparities, increased placement stability, less stigma with foster care, and preservation of sibling relationships (Cuddeback, 2004; Geen, 2004). Current best evidence suggests that children in kinship care may do better than children in traditional foster care in terms of their behavior, development, mental health functioning, and placement stability (Winokur, Holtan, & Valentine, 2009).

KINSHIP CAREGIVERS' HEALTH STATUS

Although there is evidence to support the benefits of kinship care for children, much less has been reported regarding how kinship caregivers fare. To determine how the health status of relative adoptive parents (n = 469) compared with that of nonrelative adoptive parents (n = 1,599), my colleagues and I analyzed data from the National Survey of Adoptive Parents (NSAP) to examine overall physical and emotional health status (Foli, Lim, & Sands, 2015). Remember, these are kinship parents who legally adopted their children. We found that only nonrelated mothers of children younger than 6 years reported better emotional health than those who were related to their children; with this exception, physical and emotional health status did not differ between these two groups. We also found the family is indeed a social unit, and that the level of perceived happiness in the parent–child relationship was important in terms of parental health status. Despite reporting that the children under their care had experienced more maltreatment (abuse and neglect, and exposure to drugs and alcohol), relative adoptive parents reported using fewer services than their nonrelative counterparts (Foli et al., 2015). Specific questions regarding caregiver depression, parenting stress, and caregiver burden were not included in the questions contained in the NSAP.

Elder Abuse

The statistics surrounding elder abuse, including neglect and exploitation, are striking: 1 in 10 adults, aged 60 or older and who live at home, experience elder abuse (Centers for Disease Control and Prevention, 2015). This is considered an underestimation of the magnitude of the problem. Elder abuse has several forms—from physical harm, to neglect, to financial exploitation (see Exhibit 6.1). Although we know that more often the perpetrators are family members, many APNs would not regard the children of kinship caregivers as potential abusers (Brownell & Berman, 2000; Brownell, Berman, Nelson, & Fofana, 2003).

Preservation of the family takes on new meaning when applied to a kinship family. Ethical and difficult questions arise when evidence of elder abuse surfaces: Should the child/adolescent be removed from the home and placed with a foster family (away from his or her network of extended family)? What is the balance between elder safety and the child/adolescent behaviors that may have been generated through maltreatment and trauma? Brownell and Berman (2000) stated:

> Although kinship care of dependent children is not new, the child welfare system that has evolved to date is structured to place children in traditional foster care settings and to move children who cannot return home to their biological parents as quickly as possible to permanency (usually meaning adoption). The system is traditionally child-centered. Foster parents are considered professional caregivers and are expected to maintain and meet predetermined standards as a condition of placement. Children who act out in care are moved to another foster placement. Adolescents are usually moved to congregate care facilities like group homes or into "independent living" situations. Recognizing and respecting the family preservation goal of kinship care is important in developing new program models and treatment modalities

EXHIBIT 6.1
ELDER ABUSE

The Administration on Aging defines elder abuse:

"In general, elder abuse is a term referring to any knowing, intentional, or negligent act by a caregiver or any other person that causes harm or a serious risk of harm to a vulnerable adult. Legislatures in all 50 states have passed some form of elder abuse prevention laws. Laws and definitions of terms vary considerably from one state to another, but broadly defined, abuse may be:

☐ **Physical Abuse**—*inflicting physical pain or injury on a senior, for example, slapping, bruising, or restraining by physical or chemical means.*

☐ **Sexual Abuse**—*non-consensual sexual contact of any kind.*

☐ **Neglect**—*the failure by those responsible to provide food, shelter, health care, or protection for a vulnerable elder.*

☐ **Exploitation**—*the illegal taking, misuse, or concealment of funds, property, or assets of a senior for someone else's benefit.*

☐ **Emotional Abuse**—*inflicting mental pain, anguish, or distress on an elder person through verbal or nonverbal acts, e.g., humiliating, intimidating, or threatening.*

☐ **Abandonment**—*desertion of a vulnerable elder by anyone who has assumed the responsibility for care or custody of that person.*

☐ **Self-neglect**—*characterized as the failure of a person to perform essential, self-care tasks and that such failure threatens his/her own health or safety."*

Source: Administration on Aging (2016).

that address the problem of grandparent abuse, before it becomes too serious for the adolescent to remain in the family or even the community. (p. 104)

This description of the context of elder maltreatment within the wider scope of foster care practices and trans- and intergenerational trauma is insightful. The APN will be one of the first providers to assess elder and child abuse, and will need such a context to provide patient- and family-centered care.

Military Kinship Families

A special type of kinship care revolves around military deployment. Increasingly, women are called to serve, and now, with the repeal of Title 10 U.S. Code, section 6015, women may be assigned to any combat unit, class of combat vessels, and combat platform. Since this change, women have been increasingly serving in the military, and as a result, kinship parents have been asked to assist during times of deployment.

In a descriptive study of 23 kinship parents from military deployment, Bunch, Eastman, and Moore (2007) reported that the parents experienced changes in partner relationships and social networks, and that only 35% had legal custody of the children. Of note for APNs, the majority cited a change in health status, with only 35% reporting their health status as "good" (Bunch, Eastman, & Moore, 2007). It should be noted that kinship providers in military deployment situations, as with other kinship arrangements, may be siblings, aunts, uncles, and close family friends.

Trauma-Informed Parenting

In the chapter that focused on adoptive parents, I introduced the National Child Traumatic Stress Network (NCTSN), the concept of trauma-informed parenting, and the wide range of resources available to health care providers. One resource that I have used is a curriculum specifically designed for kinship, adoptive, and foster care parents. Developed by the NCTSN, "Caring for Children Who Have Experienced Trauma" (Resource Parent Curriculum [RPC]; Grillo, 2010a, 2010b) is specifically designed for resource parents (i.e., kinship, foster, and adoptive parents). Advanced by experts from around the country, the RPC is seen as a vital resource for nonbirth parents who are caring for vulnerable children. This curriculum is *free to the public* (developed with federal funds), and is being implemented by a number of organizations (see Exhibit 6.2). The goals of this curriculum include educational information about traumatized

EXHIBIT 6.2

CARING FOR CHILDREN WHO HAVE EXPERIENCED TRAUMA: RESOURCE PARENT CURRICULUM (RPC) MODULES*

- ☐ *Module 1/Introductions: Setting the climate for the workshop, including the stories of children who have experienced trauma.*
- ☐ *Module 2/Trauma 101: Describing trauma and what can be done to help children.*
- ☐ *Module 3/Understanding Trauma's Effects: Children's developmental stages and trauma are considered.*
- ☐ *Module 4/Building a Safe Place: The concept of safety—physical and psychological— is discussed and its importance to children who have experienced trauma.*
- ☐ *Module 5/Dealing With Feelings and Behavior: How trauma translates into children's feelings and behaviors so that appropriate strategies can be formulated.*
- ☐ *Module 6/Connections and Healing: Children's connections are critical to emotional well-being, and ways to foster connections are discussed.*
- ☐ *Module 7/Becoming an Advocate: Helping RPC parents work with teams of professionals and advocate for their children is emphasized.*
- ☐ *Module 8/Taking Care of Yourself: The effects of secondary stress and trauma on the parent are described with strategies for self-care.*

*Each of the 8 modules is approximately 90 minutes in length (Grillo, Lott, Foster Care Subcommittee of the Child Welfare Committee, & National Child Traumatic Stress Network, 2010a, 2010b).

children and how to respond to challenging behaviors and emotions, as well as how caregivers can take care of themselves and seek support from others. Preliminary empirical evidence appears to support these impressions. Sullivan et al. (2016) reported that kinship parents demonstrated significantly increased knowledge related to trauma-informed care as well as self-efficacy after the RPC curriculum.

In my project, which was supported through funding from the National Institute of Food and Agriculture, we provided health education in cooperation/partnership between nursing faculty and rural-based Purdue University Extension Educators. Purdue University, as part of its land grant mission, has a network of extension educators who are cross-trained to deliver a variety of content, including human development and health and wellness. As members of the communities they serve, extension educators are in key positions to deliver the RPC to kinship parents. The stigma associated with receiving mental health services cuts across urban and rural areas; however, the familiarity that is characteristic of rural communities exacerbates this stigma and often precludes individuals from seeking much needed services. By engaging extension educators, embedding this health education within the umbrella of Purdue Extension, and partnering with nursing faculty, we strategically attempted to decrease the stigma associated with mental illness.

The RPC is unique in several key areas. First, there is an emphasis on the "why" of the child's behavior from a resource (i.e., kinship, foster, or adoptive) parent's perspective. For example, if a child demonstrates externalizing behaviors at bedtime (hiding/hoarding food), rather than thinking of consequences to extinguish the behavior, the kinship parent is encouraged to look beyond overt behaviors and attempt to ascertain what is triggering the child's need to demonstrate maladaptive coping. The child may be concerned about having adequate food upon wakening, having been traumatized by food insecurity or as a reaction to having been victimized through sexual abuse at bedtime (Reagan-Shaw, Sullivan, Sharda, Foreman, & Badeau, 2012). Second, the curriculum includes a focused application through a "My Child" worksheet that enables the kinship parent to apply the concepts of trauma-informed parenting to their child(ren). Third, there is a module devoted to "Taking Care of Yourself," during which the kinship parents learn about signs and symptoms of compassion fatigue and secondary trauma (Grillo, Lott, Foster Care Subcommittee of the Child Welfare Committee, & National Child

Traumatic Stress Network, 2010a, 2010b). Based on my professional experience, this curriculum is a powerful tool to support kinship parents' ability to not only understand trauma, but also begin to heal from its effects.

During these classes, the statistics surrounding kinship parents' struggles become more than sterile, benign numbers on a page. The parents sit, lean forward, and tell their narratives, heartbreaking stories of adult children who have become addicted to substances and are now individuals who cannot be trusted, cannot be left alone with their children. The kinship parents become protectors of the grandchildren who have come to live with them, fierce gatekeepers to prevent further maltreatment. Some confess to generational abuse they themselves have endured. I listen and wonder whether they have ever disclosed these personal traumas to another human being. I see the tears, the heads lowered in shame.

The children come in from the adjacent room where I have arranged student nurses to provide supervision. They grab snacks, handful after handful, as if they know to grab food when it is available to them. They have made craft projects and offer the completed projects to their grandparents. Later, after the children have left, we discuss what is meant by "mom" and "dad," and who says these to them. The kinship parents report discomfort at being called these titles. Still, they almost universally report that the children under their care want to call them "mom" and "dad." They make up other names, offshoots of "grandmother" and "grandfather," and insist they are not the parents. I offer that children signify who loves them, who meets their needs, and who provides safety to them by these words.

They discuss trauma, violence, neglect, physical and psychological dangers that the children—and sometimes they—have endured. Other times, the kinship caregivers relate that the birth parents simply do not know how to care for children because they are too immature to take on the responsibilities of parenthood. The birth parents are transients in the home, sometimes there and sometimes not. Their role in the child's life shifts as maturity develops. The kinship parent may find that even after years of parenting a child, they have no rights to a permanent parenting relationship when the birth parent emerges once again to assume a full-time role in the child's life.

CASE STUDIES: KINSHIP PARENTS

□ □ □ □

CASE STUDY 1: SALLY

Sally is a 68-year-old woman who has assumed the care of her 4-year-old grandson because his mother, her daughter, has been incarcerated for methamphetamine use and dealing. She is recovering postoperatively from total knee replacement surgery she had 3 days ago, and is in a subacute care rehabilitation facility for 2 weeks for physical therapy and 24-hour nursing care.

Sally has taken care of her 4-year-old grandson, Joshua, "on and off" since he was born. A widow, Sally lives in an old house, badly in need of repairs in a lower socioeconomic neighborhood. The boy's father has not contacted the family for over 2 years. While at the rehabilitation facility, Sally's friend has been looking after Joshua, but is getting tired. The caseworker from the DCS is not aware of Sally's friend caring for Joshua because Sally is worried he will end up in a foster home. She has intentionally kept DCS out of their lives because she feels so vulnerable and worried that, because of the disrepair of her home, they will take Joshua away. Her primary concern is not being able to carry food home from the food pantry once she gets home and Joshua feeling abandoned. Sally knows he starts to regress when she is sick, and this is the longest they have been apart. Her friend has complained about Joshua's bedwetting, something he had stopped a year ago with Sally.

The physical therapy has been difficult on Sally, especially with her body mass index (BMI) of under 19. But she is trying her hardest to get home. She hopes to be discharged within the next 2 days.

APN Next Steps

As Sally stands with the help of the physical therapy aide, Janet, her adult-gerontology nurse practitioner (A-GNP), walks into her room. Janet assesses Sally's circulation and watches as she ambulates from her room and down the hallway. Janet has already reviewed the medical record and seen that Sally's recovery has been fairly uneventful. The cefazolin has been effective in preventing infection, and physical therapy is proceeding smoothly. The continuous passive motion (CPM) machine is also effective, according to the electronic health record (EHR).

Janet notices a little boy entering the hallway and running up to Sally. He is clearly glad to see her and shows her a picture he has drawn. Sally strokes his brown hair and touches his cheek as she pauses from walking. The lady who brought the boy is also an older adult and looks tired and annoyed. Sally looks nervously at Janet, and shakes her head at the woman. Janet approaches a bit closer and hears Sally state, "Not now! We can talk later. You know I appreciate all you're doing."

Janet stops beside Sally and asks, "Everything okay?" Sally looks down and then at the other woman, who excuses herself and leaves. Joshua says, "Look, Grandmamma, look what I drew!"

Sally blinks and smiles, and then turns to Janet. Hanging onto the bar on the wall, Sally confides that she is taking care of the boy, her grandson, and has all his life. Her friend is helping with the child until she goes home. They arrive back at Sally's room, and Janet watches as the boy goes to Sally's lunch tray and eats the food that Sally has saved for him. Janet begins to stop him, but realizes the boy is very hungry.

Janet nods reassuringly, and knows Sally's recovery may be jeopardized without support and solid discharge planning. Janet realizes Sally is a kinship parent and extremely vulnerable for several reasons. While Sally finishes her physical therapy, Janet calls social services to discuss Sally's discharge plans. She informs the case manager of what she has learned and arranges for Sally to have a care conference, which will include taking care of an active child.

Two days later, during the case conference, with Sally present, the team discusses discharge plans. Based on Sally's income, the case manager feels that Sally is entitled to Temporary Assistance for Needy Families (TANF). In Sally's state of residence, it is possible for DCS to allow physical and legal custody of Joshua without formal foster parenting; however, additional resources would be available if Sally became Joshua's foster parent. The facility social worker has corresponded with the DCS caseworker, and they are arranging a meeting to discuss steps for Sally to become Joshua's guardian and foster mother, which would open up needed resources for the family.

Follow-Up

Janet works under a collaboration agreement with a physician and sees Sally the following week in the outpatient setting. Sally is overwhelmed by the paperwork that is required to become a foster parent, but she is slowly working through it. Janet assesses Sally's weight and notices that she has gained 2 pounds; lab work is normal with slightly elevated levels of cortisol. Janet is concerned as elevated cortisol is common following surgery, but she also knows that Sally is under significant stress as a result of taking care of an active younger child. Janet knows that the cortisol may be eating away at muscle-building protein and making her rehabilitation/mobility that much more difficult. She also knows the loss of protein means poor wound healing.

Janet discusses this finding with Sally and educates her on how to take care of herself first so that she can better meet Joshua's needs. She encourages low-resource stress relievers such as going to the library or keeping a journal; she alerts Sally to low-cost activities that she can enjoy with Joshua in the community that will also increase her mobility. Last, Janet assesses whether Sally will need a social service consult to complete the foster care paperwork so that she can obtain the resources she needs for her and Joshua.

□ □ □ □

CASE STUDY 2: SAMUEL

Samuel, or Sam, is a 56-year-old divorced man who has assumed the role of caring for his oldest daughter's children. His daughter is a single parent who has been on military deployment for several months. Sam has struggled with obesity his entire life and now feels compelled to change his habits to a healthier lifestyle. The two little boys, ages 4 and 5 years, are often more than he can handle. He has caught himself being winded after playing catch with them in the backyard, but he has been eating more for quick spurts of energy. The laundry, grocery shopping, driving the kids to sports, and being a single parent are overwhelming. He has added stress at work because of feeling pressured to leave in time to pick up the boys from day care before it closes.

Working at a desk job in data management only increases his inactivity. As a result, his blood glucose levels at home range between 212 mg/dL in the morning before breakfast and 335 mg/dL after eating. He is on antihypertensive and cardiac medications for his history of congestive heart failure, but often forgets to take his medicine. He also has a history of hyperlipidemia. He has been taking Lisinopril 10 mg daily, metformin 1,000 mg twice daily, metoprolol XL 50 mg daily, and atorvastatin 20 mg daily. He is being seen for his follow-up appointment with his primary care A-GPN, Elaine.

Samuel arrives at his scheduled appointment and is concerned when his intake weight is 250 pounds, 15 pounds more than 6 months ago. His blood pressure reading is 178/94, heart rate is 78, and his oxygen saturation rate is 94%. He feels stressed and is not sleeping well.

APN Next Steps

The A-GNP, Elaine, reviews the labs (hemoglobin A1c, fasting lipids, comprehensive metabolic panel, and microalbumin) she ordered to be drawn before today's visit. They are normal or only slightly out of the acceptable range with the exception of his hemoglobin A1c level, which is 9.2. Elaine can sense that Sam is very stressed when she enters the room. He looks fatigued, and he is only able to offer a weak smile. Elaine sits down and asks, "Tell me how you're feeling."

Sam relates how he is overeating for energy, but then has rebound low energy in the afternoon. Elaine listens and offers congruent nonverbal signals to communicate that she is listening and attentive.

"Sam, I noticed your weight was up a bit," Elaine stated.

"I know! It is just I'm a single parent now, and I was never that great of a cook so we eat fast food—a lot. Now, it's all I can do to get the boys to after-school stuff and then, there's homework." His words spill out, even in tone, but defensive.

Elaine understands that Sam is on overload, needs to breathe and take a moment to compose himself. Because Sam is in the day-to-day grind of being a single parent at the age of 56, and holding down a full-time job, she knows her best strategy is to help him find his own motivation and perspective. She reassures Sam that she is not there to chastise him in any way, and that her role is to support him in achieving health and balance in his life. She then uses motivational interviewing (Miller & Rollnick, 2004) techniques to try to help Sam find answers for himself. Her goal is to have Sam find his own motivation for change and commit to it. She uses the Socratic method so that Sam can avoid resisting changes that she may want him to make, and instead arrive at those changes through his own discovery and motivation (Miller & Rollnick, 2004).

At the end of the discussion, Sam agrees to preplan meals on Sundays and reduce eating fast foods to twice a week. He smiles as he realizes that the situation will last only until his daughter is finished with her assignment, another 6 months. He admits that there is a group of colleagues who try to walk during their lunch hours, and he has been invited to join them. His boss has offered him a standing desk so that he would not be sitting all day. He also agrees to speak to the clinic dietitian and look for ways to eat healthier alternatives. Elaine interjects that buying a water bottle with measures on the side will allow him to measure his fluid intake.

She discusses the management plan with him: increase Lisinopril to 20 mg daily, continue metformin and other medications as ordered. There will be a new medication, glyburide 2.5 mg, to be taken with breakfast; and last, she discusses the use of a selective serotonin reuptake inhibitor (SSRI) to assist in managing his stress. Elaine also instructs him on taking serial blood pressure readings at home, and emphasizes the need for him to exercise as much as possible, ideally, 20 minutes of exercise five times per week. She would like him to bring the food, exercise, blood pressure, and blood glucose logs to his next visit. Sam seems to take it all in and appears less anxious than when he arrived. Elaine asks him to return in 3 weeks for a follow-up.

□ □ □ □

CASE STUDY 3: NANCY

Nancy is a 61-year-old African American woman who has "inherited" a kinship arrangement from her second husband. The birth mother, Kandi, is in and out of the household, sometimes sleeping in their spare bedroom, sometimes out all night. Nancy's husband has been laid off, and she has been working extra hours at the retail store where she works. She takes her 4-year old granddaughter, Maxeene, to a health center clinic that distributes the Women, Infants and Children

(WIC) program cards that she can use at the grocery store. Nancy is also receiving TANF, which has qualified her to receive WIC services. The WIC nurse asks how Nancy has been getting along, and she confides in her that she has been having difficulty sleeping, and during the day, feeling very "panicky." She has also had a flare-up of her rheumatoid arthritis. The nurse makes a referral to the community mental health center for Nancy to see a psychiatric-mental health nurse practitioner (PMHNP).

Three weeks later, Nancy is evaluated by the PMHNP, Pam, who takes a full history from Nancy. Pam determines that Nancy's own upbringing was fairly chaotic, with a single parent, whose own extended family was in and out of the home, including several male figures. Nancy's panic attacks have escalated since she took in her granddaughter. Nancy begins crying as she relates that she is aware that Maxeene has been sexually and physically abused. She was present when the caseworker interviewed Maxeene, who explained her drawings of the abuse. Nancy denies that such trauma is in her history, but shares how difficult it is to know that this "little innocent soul" has experienced so much. She relates how she wishes she could help Maxeene more, but does not know how.

Nancy is hypervigilant about Maxeene, rarely letting her out of her sight. When Kandi is in the house, Nancy ensures that Maxeene is never alone with her or anyone Kandi has brought home. She obsesses about Maxeene while she is at work and makes her husband promise to "watch over her—don't take your eyes off her for a minute." The panic attacks have increased in the past few weeks with shortness of breath, agitation, and a feeling of terror.

APN Next Steps

Pam diagnoses Nancy with panic disorder (American Psychiatric Association, 2013). She explains to Nancy how caring for Maxeene has triggered some thoughts from her past and, furthermore, created secondary trauma from learning about the abuse that Maxeene has experienced. She supports Nancy as a caring and empathic grandmother who deeply wants a safe environment for Maxeene with no further abuse. Pam and Nancy begin cognitive behavioral therapy (CBT) in a partnership. The goal is to decrease Nancy's symptoms of panic disorder through challenging her patterns of catastrophizing and by practicing grounding behaviors. She is dosed with an SSRI by Pam to assist in decreasing her panic attacks and is also provided with education about its use. They also work on issues such as relationship satisfaction and feeling safe.

Maxeene is referred to a child therapist with training and experience in working with children who have survived sexual abuse. This therapist includes play therapy and provides education to Nancy and her husband at the end of the child's appointment. She also works with Nancy to set boundaries and obtain legal guardianship.

Three months later, Nancy reports a decrease in her feelings of panic. She now has insight into how her past influenced her ability to parent Maxeene effectively. Her goals are being achieved with the use of therapy and psychopharmacological interventions. Nancy and her husband are able to have "date nights" with a trusted babysitter, Nancy's friend. Nancy and her friend have a barter system arranged and exchange doing "favors" with one another (e.g., cooking meals, babysitting, rides to appointments). Both Nancy and Maxeene continue with their treatment plans and continue to see gains in their health status.

□ □ □ □

CASE STUDY 4: MARGARET

Margaret is a 70-year-old great-grandmother to her 13-year-old kinship child, Lisa. Margaret is a widow to Ralph, who passed away 2 years ago, about the same time that Lisa came to live with her. Together they live in a rural county and seek health care primarily when a condition has advanced to the point they can no longer manage it. They consider folks who do not live in the county outsiders who will need to earn the trust of people who have resided in the area, often for generations. Margaret has a secret: Lisa punches her with her fists when Lisa becomes agitated, especially in the evenings at bedtime. Margaret is a petite woman who barely reaches 110 pounds, whereas Lisa is a "big-boned" child and already weighs 130 pounds. Lisa also plays soccer at the local middle school and is the team captain. Before coming to live with Margaret, Lisa witnessed significant domestic violence between her parents who are in jail for charges related to drug use and dealing. Past traumatic events also include seeing her parents handcuffed in front of her when she was only 8 years old.

Lisa loves Margaret and is good to her most of the time. However, Lisa cannot control her anger and has been physically abusive for 2 years. In Lisa's tirades, she blames Margaret for the loss of her parents, "If you had been a better parent the first time, my parents wouldn't have turned to drugs." Margaret tries to defend herself, but has become increasingly depressed, with marked weight loss and neglect of personal appearance and hygiene.

Lisa is careful to only punch Margaret in the back and abdomen, so the bruises do not show. Margaret has withdrawn from church and other social activities as Lisa's aggression has grown. After one particularly violent exchange, Margaret wakes up one morning unable to move her left arm. Significant swelling above her elbow, where Lisa yanked her the previous evening, is also evident.

After she hears Lisa leave for school, Margaret reluctantly drives herself to the city about 30 miles away to the emergency department. She completes the intake form as best she can, stating that her arm was injured because she fell down the basement stairs and caught herself on the railing, which injured her arm. She is nervous and in significant pain. She has not eaten since last night, and only had a few bites as she is struggling to keep enough food in the house for both her and Lisa. Finally, Margaret is told she will be seen and is escorted to a patient room.

She sits on a bed, not wanting to disrobe for fear that the new and healing bruising on her torso will be revealed. After a few minutes, a medical technician comes in to take her blood pressure, temperature, pulse rate, and oxygen saturation level through a finger pulse oximeter. She also asks Margaret for a brief history of the injury, and she conveys her story about almost falling down the basement stairs.

The technician leaves, and after a few minutes, Margaret sees a woman, about 30 years of age, enter the room. She introduces herself as Jean, an emergency department nurse practitioner (ENP) who will be assessing her.

APN Next Steps

Jean notes Margaret's nervous affect and how she is hugging her torso with her right arm. The left arm has been immobilized with an old towel. She sees a disheveled older adult whose vital signs are stable with the exception of a lower oxygen saturation of 92%. Jean knows this could be due to shallow breathing resulting from pain, and performs a pain assessment. She asks Margaret to give her a number, between 1 and 10 (the Numeric Rating Scale) of any pain she is currently experiencing. Jean also asks what her normal level of comfort is. Margaret hesitates, but the pain is increasing, and rates her arm pain at 9 out of 10.

Jean gently removes the towel from around the right arm and notes swelling in the proximal area of the humerus near the shoulder. Jean checks for peripheral pulses and sensation of feeling in the affected extremity. In consultation with her collaborating physician, she orders an x-ray of the arm and includes anterior/posterior, transscapular, and axillary views. This will determine whether there is a proximal humeral fracture, fairly common in women, especially those with osteoporosis, and any displacement of the bone. But there is something bothering Jean about Margaret, and her story of catching herself before she fell.

Although Jean does not want to move Margaret unnecessarily, she feels that the assessment is not complete. Wanting to ensure that respiratory status is not compromised, she tells Margaret that she would like to listen to her lungs before they take her to x-ray. Margaret bites her lip and nods. As Jean lifts Margaret's shirt in the back, she notes significant contusions in various stages of resolution with colors, including yellow-brown, and blue-green bruising of the skin.

Jean listens to Margaret's lungs and instructs her to take deep breaths, which she is unable to do because of pain. Jean gently replaces Margaret's shirt and sits beside her. Jean knows that establishing trust and rapport is critical to understanding what the patient has experienced. If she comes on too strong, and begins an "interrogation"-type interview, Margaret is likely to shut down.

Jean states, "I used to live in the country. I really enjoyed the beauty of nature and the seasons."

"Yes. We really like it." Margaret does not make eye contact.

"I read on your intake that you have a 13-year-old granddaughter who lives with you."

"Yes. She's a good girl."

Jean uses silence for a few seconds. "Margaret, let's review how you hurt your arm." For the next few minutes, Jean collects information about the current injury. She finally states, "I see. But I also noticed there are several areas on your back that have been injured."

Margaret looks down, but does not respond.

Jean relaxes her posture, but leans slightly forward. "I'm concerned about you and these injuries. This must be hard to hear, but if someone is hurting you, you can tell me. I know this is hard to talk about."

Margaret finally looks at Jean and in a whisper says, "It's my granddaughter, Lisa. I'm afraid of her. She hits me with her fists and it hurts. Sometimes, it really hurts. She's been through so much, though, you know. With her parents. Sometimes, she blames me." Tears roll down Margaret's cheeks; she continues to look at Jean for her reactions.

"It must have been hard for you to tell me this. I want you to know that it's brave to be able to talk about this." Jean discusses the interactions between Margaret and Lisa and collects more information. She realizes that the family is in crisis in several areas: social, financial, emotional, and physical. She watches Margaret as she leaves for radiology, and discusses what she has uncovered with the collaborating physician. They file a report with Adult Protective Services and offer information pertaining to Margaret's case. X-rays reveal that Margaret's fracture will be treated without surgery, and the limb is immobilized. Margaret refuses other services before leaving the emergency department.

Caseworkers investigate the report by sending a social worker to the home within 24 hours to determine Margaret's safety and

TABLE 6.2   *Kinship Parents: What to Look for and What to Do*

Kinship Parents

What to Look for (Assessment):

☐ Assess for safety issues within the family, including signs and symptoms of both child and elder abuse, and report this information.

☐ Assess for caregiver burden and older adult depressive symptoms using validated screening tools.

☐ Monitor for signs of psychological distress, including compassion fatigue, depression, and chronic stress.

☐ Monitor for signs and symptoms of chronic disease exacerbations, which may be related to mental health issues (e.g., depression, stress, or caregiver burden).

(continued)

TABLE 6.2   *Kinship Parents: What to Look for and What to Do (continued)*

What to Do (Management):
- ☐ Ensure chronic diseases are monitored and managed.
- ☐ Reduce stigma and guilt by providing psychosocial support and therapeutic communication.
- ☐ Refer questions related to guardianship, foster care, and legal adoption to social workers, case managers, and adoption-competent attorneys.
- ☐ Refer to social workers to optimize financial and social support as appropriate.
- ☐ Provide trauma-informed care, understanding that trauma in some kinship families is multigenerational.
- ☐ Promote self-efficacy and resourcefulness through the use of feedback and evidence-based interventions, such as journaling.

well-being. She then arranges for Margaret to receive much needed services, including TANF, relative caregiver state subsidies, family counseling, and individual counseling for both Margaret and Lisa. Safety follow-up for Margaret will be a priority.

APNs' CARE OF KINSHIP PARENTS

Kinship parents differ in significant ways from traditional foster care parents, and present with both challenges and strengths. Unique to kinship providers are the chronic illnesses that require the APN to monitor and manage. These may be adversely affected by caregiver burden, depressive symptoms, parental stress, and compassion fatigue. APNs will need to be sensitive to those kinship caregivers who remain "off the grid" from government systems, such as child welfare agencies, and will need to refer to much needed resources. Research supports that these parents need services, but often access fewer than traditional foster parents. Thus, the skilled APN will need to persuade, motivate, and negotiate so that the kinship family receives the needed financial and social supports (Table 6.2).

CHAPTER HIGHLIGHTS

- ☐ In general, kinship parents are an at-risk population with their own health care needs, limited financial resources, and preoccupation with caring for children who have often experienced maltreatment.
- ☐ Kinship families may be categorized by types, with the largest class, "empty-nest grandparents," most likely to experience health problems.

☐ Caregiving grandmothers often experience depression, stress, and interfamily strain.

☐ Kinship parents may experience compassion fatigue, acute stress disorder, secondary trauma, or posttraumatic stress disorder associated with caring for their children.

☐ Benefits to the children in kinship care versus traditional foster care are well documented and include: behavior, development, mental health functioning, and placement stability.

☐ Elder abuse is growing and includes both abuse and neglect; kinship caregivers may be at risk for maltreatment from both adult children and the children under their care.

Questions for Reflection

Following are a few questions to reflect upon. You can use these to start a journal for yourself or in a classroom discussion with peers and the instructor.

1. Have you or has someone you know acted as a kinship parent? What were the needs of the kinship caregiver? How could an APN contribute to positive outcomes?
2. What stigma do you associate with kinship parenting? What constitutes a "good parent"? Where does parent culpability lie in offspring who abuse alcohol and illegal substances?
3. What policies/legislation should the United States consider to promote the well-being of kinship parents?
4. How can resources reach kinship providers who prefer to remain "off the grid," with no contact with the Department of Child Services/Child Welfare?
5. Have you rendered care to an older adult who may have been the victim of elder abuse? How did you handle the situation? To whom did you report the abuse?
6. What case study spoke to you the most? Why? What personal and professional feelings were evoked within you?

References

Administration on Aging. (2016). Retrieved from www.aoa.acl.gov/AoA_Programs/Elder_Rights/EA_Prevention/whatIsEA.aspx

American Psychiatric Association. (2013). *Diagnostic and statistical manual of mental disorders* (5th ed.). Arlington, VA: American Psychiatric Publishing.

Annie E. Casey Foundation. (2012). *Stepping up for kids: What government and communities should do to support kinship families.* Baltimore, MD: Author.

Baum, L. F. (1900). *The wizard of Oz.* London, England: Penguin Books.

Brownell, P., & Berman, J. (2000). Risks of caregiving: Abuse within the relationship. In C. B. Cox (Ed.), *To grandmother's house we go. . .and stay: Perspectives on custodial grandparents* (pp. 91–109). New York, NY: Springer Publishing.

Brownell, P., Berman, J., Nelson, A., & Fofana, R. C. (2003). Grandparents raising grandchildren: The risks of caregiving. *Journal of Elder Abuse and Neglect, 15*(3-4), 5–31. doi:10.1300/j084v15n03_02

Bunch, S. G., Eastman, B. J., & Moore, R. R. (2007). A profile of grandparents raising grandchildren as a result of parental military deployment. *Journal of Human Behavior in the Social Environment, 15*(4), 1–12. doi:10.1300/J137v15n04_01

Centers for Disease Control and Prevention. (2015). Elder abuse prevention. Retrieved from www.cdc.gov/features/elderabuse/

ChildFocus® & The North American Council on Adoptable Children. (2010). Kinship adoption: Meeting the unique needs of a growing population. Retrieved from childfocuspartners.com/wp-content/uploads/CF_Kinship_Adoption_Report_v5.pdf

Child Welfare Information Gateway. (2016). *Foster care statistics 2014.* Washington, DC: U.S. Department of Health and Human Services, Children's Bureau.

Cuddeback, G. S. (2004). Kinship family foster care: A methodological and substantive synthesis of research. *Children and Youth Services Review, 26,* 623–639.

Foli, K. J., Lim, E., & Sands, L. P. (2015). Comparison of relative and non-relative adoptive parent health status. *Western Journal of Nursing Research, 37*(3), 320–341. doi:10.1177/0193945913511708

Geen, R. (2004). The evolution of kinship care policy and practice. *Children, Families, and Foster Care, 14*(1), 130–149.

Grillo, C. A., Lott, D.A., Foster Care Subcommittee of the Child Welfare Committee, & National Child Traumatic Stress Network. (2010a). *Caring for children who have experienced trauma: A workshop for resource parents— Facilitator's guide.* Los Angeles, CA & Durham, NC: National Center for Child Traumatic Stress.

Grillo, C. A., Lott, D.A., Foster Care Subcommittee of the Child Welfare Committee, & National Child Traumatic Stress Network. (2010b). *Caring for children who have experienced trauma: A workshop for resource parents—Participant handbook.* Los Angeles, CA & Durham, NC: National Center for Child Traumatic Stress.

Miller, W. R., & Rollnick, S. (2004). Talking oneself into change: Motivational interviewing, stages of change, and therapeutic process. *Journal of Cognitive Psychotherapy, 18*(4), 299–308.

Musil, C., Warner, C., Zauszniewski, J., Wykle, M., & Standing, T. (2009). Grandmother caregiving, family stress and strain, and depressive symptoms. *Western Journal of Nursing Research, 31,* 389–408. doi:10.1177/0193945908328262

Musil, C. M., Gordon, N. L., Warner, C. B., Zauszniewski, J. A., Standing, T., & Wykle, M. (2010). Grandmothers and caregiving to grandchildren: Continuity, change, and outcomes over 24 months. *The Gerontologist, 51*(1), 86–100. doi:10.1093/geront/gnq0612012

Musil, C. M., Jeanblanc, A. B., Burant, C. J., Zauszniewski, J. A., & Warner, C. B. (2013). Longitudinal analysis of resourcefulness, family strain, and depressive symptoms in grandmother caregivers. *Nursing Outlook, 61*(4), 225–234. doi:10.1016/j.outlook.2013.04.009

Musil, C. M., Zauszniewski, J. A., Burant, C. J., Toly, V. B., & Warner, C. B. (2015). Evaluating an online resourcefulness training intervention pilot test using six critical parameters. The *International Journal of Aging and Human Development, 82*(1), 117–135. doi:10.1177/0091415015623552

Reagan-Shaw, S., Sullivan, K., Sharda, E., Foreman, C., & Badeau, S. (2012, October 26). Getting started with the NCTSN Resource Parent Curriculum, or what's in it for me? [Webinar]. Retrieved from learn.nctsn.org/course/view.php?id=67

Sakai, C., Lin, H., & Flores, G. (2011). Health outcomes and family services: Analysis of a national sample of children in the child welfare system. *Archives of Pediatric and Adolescent Medicine, 165*(2), 159–165.

Sullivan, K. M., Murray, K. J., & Ake III, G. S. (2016). Trauma-informed care for children in the child welfare system: An initial evaluation of a trauma-informed parenting workshop. *Child Maltreatment, 21*(2), 147–155. doi:10.1177/1077559515615961

United States Department of Agriculture: Economic Research Service. (2015). Food security in the U.S. Retrieved from www.ers.usda.gov/topics/food-nutrition-assistance/food-security-in-the-us/key-statistics-graphics.aspx#householdtype

Vandivere, S., Malm, K., & Radel, L. (2009). *Adoption USA: A chartbook based on the 2007 National Survey of Adoptive Parents.* Washington, D.C.: The U.S. Department of Health and Human Services, Office of the Assistant Secretary for Planning and Evaluation.

Winokur, M., Holtan, A., & Valentine, D. (2009). Kinship care for the safety, permanency, and well-being of children removed from the home for maltreatment. *Campbell Systematic Reviews,* 1. doi:10.4073/csr.2009.1

Zauszniewski, J. A., Musil, C. M., Burant, C. J., & Au, T-Y. (2014). Resourcefulness training for grandmothers: Preliminary evidence of effectiveness. *Research in Nursing & Health, 37,* 42–52. doi:10.1002/nur.21574

Zinn, A. (2010). A typology of kinship foster families: Latent class and exploratory analyses of kinship family structure and household composition. *Children and Youth Services Review, 32,* 325–337. doi:10.1016/j.childyouth.2009.10.001

7

Birth Parents of Kinship Children

□ □ □ □

PURPOSE OF THE CHAPTER

Parents of children in kinship care perhaps carry the most pronounced stigma of any birth parent group. Based on the level of involvement with the Department of Child Services (DCS) and/or courts, and their relationship with the kinship caregiver, birth parents' presence in the home will vary from being a coparent to being absent from the household, often because of incarceration. The consistency of this presence influences the family system and has consequences for children, kinship parents, and birth parents. In this chapter, we explain and explore the complex and diverse relationships that exist among birth parents, their children, and the kinship caregivers who have stepped in as surrogate parents.

In our first case study, we explore the devastation caused by substance abuse with an opioid-dependent mother of three young children who struggles to regain her life. The second case describes a young mother who is in and out of the multigenerational home where her child resides. Next, we discuss a middle-aged man who has been diagnosed with stage IV lung cancer and is in hospice care. Finally, a young mother who has neither the resources nor the maturity to raise her children is described. Each of these cases represents opportunities for advanced practice nurses (APNs) to accurately assess health issues and render comfort and care.

Learning Objectives

At the completion of the chapter, the reader will be able to:

1. Describe the variations in interactions between birth parents, kinship parents, and the children

2. Analyze trends in child maltreatment in the United States from 2000 to 2010
3. Understand the ramifications of the Fostering Connections to Success and Increasing Adoptions Act of 2008 and the Child Abuse Prevention and Treatment Reauthorization Act of 2010 to birth parents in kinship families
4. Analyze the effects of substance abuse disorder on birth parents and their children's lives
5. Describe the trends in incarcerated parents and their children across the past decade
6. Synthesize the effects across generations of acute, chronic, and complex trauma

BIRTH PARENT INVOLVEMENT IN KINSHIP FAMILIES

I have conceptualized the involvement of birth parents in a continuum from coparenting to an absence from the family (see Figure 7.1). Variables that affect this continuum are whether the kinship/grandparent has established guardianship, foster parenting, or legal adoption. The family system dynamics, which are affected by legal arrangements, child welfare involvement, the presence of active substance use, and mental health issues, will influence how much presence the birth parent has—or is allowed to have—in the child's life.

In a study conducted in California, researchers examined the interactions between birth parents and 351 custodial grandmothers raising school-aged children (Green & Goodman, 2010). The researchers found

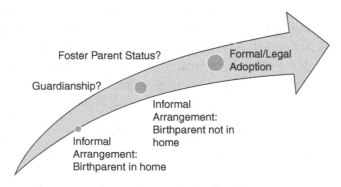

FIGURE 7.1   *Kinship care continuum.*

three groups of birth parents: high involvement (30%); moderate involvement (35%); and low involvement (35%). Birth parents were twice as likely to have high involvement in informal kinship arrangements when compared with moderate- to low-involvement groups. Other factors that contributed to high birth parent involvement included a close relationship between the birth parent and the grandparent, and the grandmother's satisfaction with life. Last, the odds of more birth parent involvement increased when the child was younger, and there was no child protective service involvement (Green & Goodman, 2010).

PARENTING AND THE LAW

The intersection of private family and the legalities of child protection is apparent when birth parents, their children, and kinship care providers are discussed. Indeed, the legal term *parens patriae* asserts that the government has the responsibility to intervene in cases where individuals cannot protect themselves, and where children may be maltreated (abused or neglected) by their parents, legal guardians, or caretakers. Because parents are no longer able or are unwilling to provide a safe and caring home for their children, kinship providers are asked to come forward. The tension between reunification with parents and their children versus permanent placement with a new family is an underlying, pervasive theme. The first federal law of note was the Adoptions and Safe Families Act of 1997 (P.L. 105-89), which shortened the time frame for the child's first permanency hearing, thus decreasing the time a child spends waiting in foster care without the opportunity to be placed in a permanent family—and shortening the time within which the child may be reunified with birth parents.

Second, the Fostering Connections to Success and Increasing Adoptions Act of 2008, signed into law by President George W. Bush, signaled changes to the child welfare system, primarily to Title IV-E of the Social Security Act. Title IV-E covers federal payments to states for foster care and adoption assistance. Of note, this historic law included provisions to keep sibling groups together and to allow states the option to provide kinship guardianship payments or payments to relative foster parents. Thus, kinship care was encouraged and supported, and birth parents' presence in the home became fluid and dependent on circumstances influenced by legal as well as family preferences.

The third important federal law is the Child Abuse Prevention and Treatment Act (CAPTA), which was initially passed in 1974 (P.L. 93-247), and most recently updated by the CAPTA Reauthorization Act of 2010 (P.L. 111-320) (Child Welfare Information Gateway, 2011). This important law provides federal resources to states for child abuse prevention and treatment. These funds include support for data collection activities, demonstration projects, services, and research grants. The APN should be aware of the strong influences these federal laws have on state practices in cases of birth parent rights and kinship families, influences that affect the health care system.

In one of the exercises in the trauma-informed parenting classes, a curriculum developed by the National Child Traumatic Stress Network, we look at the birth parent's trauma, which is described in the case study. In the exercise, empathy is felt toward the children, then the kinship/grandmother, then the foster caregiver. No one initially feels compassion toward the birth parent because in the scenario, she misses phone calls and visits with the children, creating chaos and more pain for those involved. The facilitator then draws attention to the birth parent and the reasons why the contacts were missed. One of the most striking comments I hear when teaching the classes is the disclosure from the kinship/grandparents that they now realize how their children (parents of the grandchildren) were traumatized. The understanding of multigenerational trauma is the beginning of moving forward with insight, compassion, and the potential for healing.

CHILD MALTREATMENT

CAPTA Reauthorization Act of 2010 (P.L. 111-320) defines child abuse and neglect at the federal level:

> Any recent act or failure to act on the part of a parent or caretaker, which results in death, serious physical or emotional harm, sexual abuse, or exploitation, or an act or failure to act which presents an imminent risk of serious harm.

There were 742,000 children who suffered from maltreatment in 2011. Between 2000 and 2010, the substantiated reports of child maltreatment declined; however, unsubstantiated claims increased by 16% (Conn et al., 2013; see Figure 7.2). Yet these statistics offer

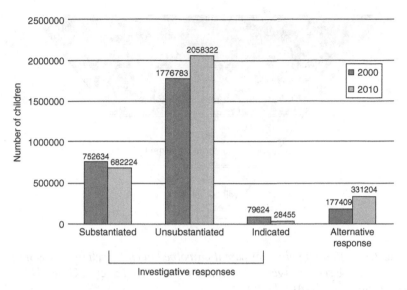

FIGURE 7.2   *Child maltreatment in the United States: 2000 to 2010.*
Source: Conn, Szilagyi, Franke, Albertin, Blumkin, and Szilagyi (2013).
Reproduced with permission from the American Academy of Pediatrics.

an incomplete picture of disturbing trends for us as a society: Over the past decade, children in out-of-home (OOH) care have a greater history of trauma, more complex needs, and current emotional disturbance when compared with OOH care in the past. Conn and colleagues (2013) concluded that these data may underestimate the needs of these vulnerable groups of children. As health care professionals, APNs are mandatory reporters of child maltreatment. The standard most often used for mandatory reporting is when the individual suspects or has reason to believe a child has been maltreated (abused or neglected; Child Welfare Information Gateway, 2016).

SUBSTANCE ABUSE

A national health crisis, substance use disorders are receiving federal government attention and resources to stem this growing problem. Birth parents whose children are in the child welfare system are frequently addicted to illegal substances. Between 50% and 80% of child welfare cases are estimated to involve parental substance abuse (Young, Boles, & Otero, 2007). As Figure 7.3 depicts, only 13 of 100 parents who are required to undergo substance abuse treatment will

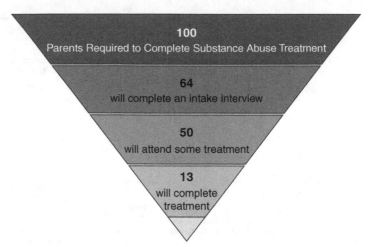

FIGURE 7.3 *Drop-off points for parents involved in child welfare accessing substance abuse services (generated from a report from the U.S. General Accounting Office [GAO] Data).*
Source: Oliveros and Kaufman (2011). Reprinted by permission.

actually complete it, whereas the majority of parents are deemed noncompliant with their case plan (Oliveros & Kaufman, 2011).

The experiences of those who are addicted and have lost custody are enlightening and need to be considered by the APN. Haight, Carter-Black, and Sheridan (2009) interviewed four rural-dwelling women who had lost their children because of substance use. The mothers described their obsession with the drug, being motivated to regain custody of their children or the threat of prison to try to end the substance use, and reliance on mothers and grandmothers to help with parenting their children. When they quit using substances, they expressed how quickly the feelings of pain and guilt would envelop them. Last, they described how quickly the addiction overcame them and became the most important thing in their lives, even more important than their children (Haight et al., 2009).

Several approaches to treat substance abuse in parents whose children are in the child welfare system were reviewed by Oliveros and Kaufman (2011). These approaches included Project SAFE (Substance Abuse Family Evaluation), motivational interviewing, Engaging Moms (EM) program, recovery coaches, family treatment drug courts, (FTDC), and home-based substance abuse interventions

(Building Stronger Families [BSF] and Family-Based Recovery [FBR]). Home-based substance abuse interventions provide intense support for the parents in the home and assist in overcoming challenges often faced by individuals, such as transportation and limited phone access (Oliveros & Kaufman, 2011). The authors call for increased research in these areas, but have concluded that FTDC and home-based substance abuse treatment interventions appear to be the most effective (Oliveros & Kaufman, 2011). A recent study described the impact of a statewide interagency cooperative program (New Jersey Child Protection Substance Abuse Initiative [CPSAI]) that showed promise in supporting birth parent treatment completion (Traube, He, Zhu, Scalise, & Richardson, 2015). Child welfare caseworkers collaborated closely with substance abuse treatment professionals to meet the parents' needs. Based on these findings, coordinating social service agency efforts support parents' attempts to overcome addiction.

When approaching parental substance abuse, it is important to strike a balance between supporting reunification efforts and ensuring the safety and well-being of the child. Currently, states vary in regard to how they approach a birth mother who is abusing substances, from assisting in obtaining treatment to prosecution and incarceration. Critics of prosecuting pregnant women who are abusing substances insist this only motivates them to hide their use and avoid treatment. Health care providers, aware of states' insistence on prosecution, may avoid reporting known instances of maternal substance abuse. In an Open Letter to the Media and Policy Makers Regarding Alarmist and Inaccurate Reporting on Prescription Opioid Use By Pregnant Women (Abrahams et al., 2013), the nonprofit group, National Advocates for Pregnant Women, calls for substance abuse to be treated as a health care issue in order to avoid "misguided policies that focus on reporting women to child welfare and law enforcement agencies for a treatable health problem that can and should be addressed through the health care system" (p. 5).

APNs can impact the lives of pregnant and postpartum women who are struggling with substance abuse by avoiding judgment and biased care, reframing substance abuse as a health problem, not a criminal act, and providing competent care in addiction treatment with a collaborating physician and a referral network of substance abuse treatment programs. To provide competent care, APNs may access toll-free, telephone consultations with physicians, clinical pharmacists, and nurses who are experts in substance use assessment and management. In partnership with the Health Resources and Services Administration (HRSA), Centers for Disease Control and Prevention (CDC), AIDS Education and Training Centers (AETC), the University of California, San Francisco (UCSF), and UCSF Department of Family and Community Medicine, the Clinical Consultation Center has been established. In addition to daytime consultations for substance use disorders, HIV/AIDS management is also available (University of California, San Francisco, 2016, nccc.ucsf.edu/clinician-consultation/substance-use-management).

INCARCERATED BIRTH PARENTS

Between 1991 and 2007, there was a 79% increase in both mothers and fathers in prison, with 62% of incarcerated women having children (Glaze & Maruschak, 2010). In 2007, combining both state and federal inmates, 2.3% or 1,706,600 U.S. children under 18 years were found to have parents who were incarcerated (Glaze & Maruschak, 2010; see Figure 7.4). Women are more likely than men to be incarcerated because of a drug offense, and 60% of mothers who are incarcerated

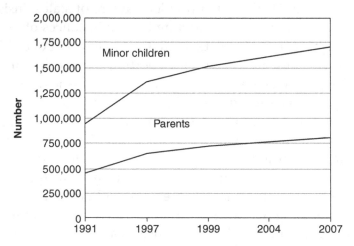

FIGURE 7.4 *Estimated number of parents in state and federal prisons and their minor children.*

Source: Glaze and Maruschak (2010).

have a history of drug dependence (The Sentencing Project, 2007). Maternal grandmothers are the most likely caregivers to children whose mothers are incarcerated (Glaze & Maruschak, 2010; The Sentencing Project, 2007; Smith, Krisman, Strozier, & Marley, 2004). Significant barriers to coparenting include physical distance and communications to update mothers on their children's status. Gaps in data are also noted as updated figures on incarcerated parents are needed to understand whether the troubling increases in parental incarceration have continued since 2007.

In a qualitative study, Strozier, Armstrong, Skuza, Cecil, and McHale (2011) interviewed 24 incarcerated mothers and 24 grandmothers who were rendering care to children between 2 and 6 years old. Two overriding themes were derived from the narratives: solidarity in parenting and an absence of solidarity, each characterizing the interactions between the birth parents and the kinship grandparents. Subthemes when solidarity was reported included compromise, shared parenting, good communication, teamwork, and similar parenting philosophies. In contrast, those parents who described a lack of solidarity also reported conflict over quality parenting, disputes over discipline, birth mother being disconnected from parenting, and despondency, guilt, and fear (Strozier et al., 2011).

CASE STUDIES: KINSHIP BIRTH PARENTS

□ □ □ □

CASE STUDY 1: MELANIE

Melanie is a 32-year-old mother of three young children (ages 5, 7, and 9 years), who has been in a residential rehabilitation substance abuse program for 4 months. She hopes to be reunited with her children, who have been cared for by her mother and stepfather. Melanie knows she is fortunate in many ways to not be incarcerated for her substance abuse. It all began 4 years ago, when she and her husband were driving home from a "date night" and were hit by a drunk driver in a car accident in which her husband was killed. With three small children to care for, Melanie's back, injured in the accident, was never allowed to heal. As her pain increased, she began taking prescription opioid medications, which she soon became dependent on.

Her physician, concerned about her increasing tolerance, refused to continue to fill the prescription. And, unable to control the cravings or afford to fill the prescription, Melanie turned to heroin. Fortunately, her parents staged an intervention, and she was given the choice of losing her children permanently or going to rehabilitation. She opted for drug treatment rehabilitation, using her husband's life insurance benefits to finance the cost. Now, 4 months later, Melanie is being seen as an outpatient by her psychiatric mental health nurse practitioner (PMHNP), Sara. Melanie was discharged from residential rehabilitation services 2 weeks before she began seeing Sara, and has been living with her mother, stepfather, and three children.

Reintegration has been stressful as each of Melanie's children processed her separation differently. Her 9-year-old son, Joe, has had the most difficult time, blaming Melanie for being absent from the family. Melanie's mother has carried the brunt of anger from Joe, who is still grieving the loss of his father, and has been irritable with Melanie since her return home. Melanie is looking for work as the financial strain on her parents has been significant. They hesitated to use Melanie's late husband's life insurance money to help her "drug problem." There is a small sum left, and her parents hoped that she could use it to "get on her feet again" with her children. The two younger children are clingy and emotionally labile, quickly changing from tears to laughter. Melanie's stepfather has become disengaged, not communicating with the family, and staying longer at work.

Melanie is also experiencing physical problems such as fatigue, joint pain, and feeling achy, with increasing back pain. She reports, when asked, that she shared needles when she was using heroin. She admits to feeling depressed and anxious.

APN Next Steps: Sara

Melanie presents to Sara, a PMHNP, as a 32-year-old female who reports feeling anxious and is slowly transitioning back into "her family." After listening to Melanie's symptoms, Sara prescribes duloxetine, which is indicated for both depression and anxiety. The APN has noticed duloxetine appears to have properties for pain relief in some of her patients and educates Melanie about potential side effects to the medication. Melanie also reports the intense cravings have increased as her stress has increased. Her guilt is overwhelming, and although she has processed much of the trauma from her husband's death, her children's trauma has renewed her memories from the night of the accident. Sara understands how at risk Melanie is to recidivism right now.

She encourages Melanie to attend the court-ordered Narcotics Anonymous (NA) meetings on a daily basis (www.na.org; see Figure 7.5). Sara describes data collected by NA in 2013 that demonstrated improvement in family relationships and social connections. More importantly, she advises Melanie to find an NA meeting that she is comfortable with, because each meeting is influenced by those who attend and what their needs might be. Sara conveys that NA, modeled after the Alcoholics Anonymous 12 steps, is a global organization with approximately 63,000 meetings each week in 132 countries across the world (NA, 2006/2014). Sara encourages Melanie's family to find support through family meetings, such as those offered through Nar-Anon.

Sara also ensures that Melanie is referred to a therapist to continue the work that was accomplished during her drug treatment inpatient stay. The therapist will begin with individual one-on-one sessions, and then determine when family therapy can be initiated because

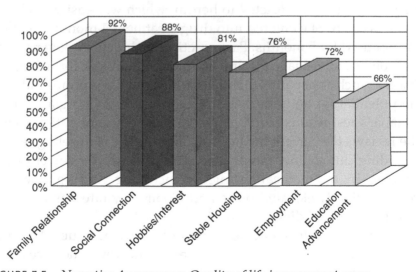

FIGURE 7.5 *Narcotics Anonymous: Quality of life improvement areas.*
Source: Reprinted by permission of NA World Services, Inc. All rights reserved.

all members of the family will need to heal from past traumas. The children will need to process their grief, including anger. Melanie's mother and stepfather will need to be included in the family therapy sessions. Sara commends Melanie on her strength and conveys that it must be difficult.

Melanie states, "I did a lot of things wrong, but I'm trying to fix them."

Sara listens as Melanie relates that her guilt has only grown worse since seeing and hearing the pain her children express. "It would be so easy to start using again. But this time, I have even more to lose. I know I'd never get them back."

Sara is concerned about Melanie's other symptoms and decides to refer Melanie to an internal medicine physician and the adult gerontology nurse practitioner (A-GNP) who practice in the clinic. Sara would like to rule out diseases such as hepatitis C and HIV as well as other infectious processes.

APN Next Steps: Georgia

Georgia is an A-GNP who has worked with her collaborating physician for 5 years. She is seeing Melanie today, a mother of three young children whose husband was killed by an intoxicated driver 4 years ago. Owing to opioid dependence/substance use, the patient became addicted to heroin, which was easier to obtain and less costly. She entered into drug treatment 4 months ago and has not used for 5 months. Past practices included sharing needles with other individuals, placing Melanie at high risk for infectious diseases such as hepatitis C and HIV. Melanie's symptoms indicate the potential for an underlying disease process. Georgia reviews Melanie's test results before entering into the examination room. She reviews the current medication list from the counseling center, including duloxetine. Finally, Georgia reviews the current data obtained by the medical technician, including vital signs, which indicate slightly elevated pulse and respiratory rates, as well as a blood pressure reading of 135/85.

Georgia introduces herself and notes how fatigued Melanie appears. The patient also has a flat affect; however, her eyes dart around the room, indicating anxiety.

Melanie blurts out: "Am I going to die?"

Georgia sits beside Melanie and relays to her that her HIV test was negative. Melanie lets out a long breath and murmurs, "Thank, God. Thank, God."

Sara waits. Melanie wipes her hand across her face and looks at Sara, who continues.

"However, your tests revealed that there is something going on that explains your symptoms of fatigue and joint pain. You've tested positive for hepatitis C virus (HCV) infection."

Melanie quickly asks, "What does this mean? Is it treatable?"

Georgia reviews the treatment options that she and her collaborating physician discussed earlier when they reviewed the patients who would be seen that day. She discusses that liver function tests will need to be ordered and that Melanie will be referred to an infectious disease specialist for the most current treatments for acute HCV infections. She asks Melanie whether duloxetine has been effective, and informs her that on the basis of the liver function tests, she may need to be changed to another antidepressant medication.

Georgia senses that Melanie is shutting down. "Is there someone with you today?"

Melanie replies that her mother is in the waiting room. Georgia places her hand on Melanie's arm. "I understand this is a lot to take in."

After Melanie looks at Georgia, the A-GNP continues to educate Melanie about how the disease is transmitted and the precautions she needs to take. Melanie nods, "I guess it's God's way of punishing me for all I've done."

Georgia looks at Melanie, "You feel you somehow deserve this?"

She shrugs her shoulders. "Yeah. I kinda do. But at least I don't have AIDS."

Georgia leans forward to meet Melanie's eyes. "I believe that things happen to people— good people and people who stumble at times. And I know that we all try to cope with what happens in our lives. One thing I believe is that a higher being—God, if you will—doesn't punish us. We often punish ourselves. I hope you know that there's much we can do to help you control this disease."

Melanie seems relieved and manages to smile.

"Now, let's talk about your back pain." Georgia performs a pain assessment. She understands that the chronic back pain can be exacerbated by depression and anxiety, but that in Melanie's case, caution and thoughtfulness need to be used to avoid recidivism. Georgia explains complementary and alternative medicine (CAM) techniques, such as acupuncture, that are used to control pain. She refers Melanie to a CAM specialist whom the practice often uses. Melanie takes the information and thanks Georgia. She leaves the office with the referral information and her mother, still overwhelmed, but with a management plan in place.

□ □ □ □

Case Study 2: Hope

Hope is a 19-year-old African American woman, living with her grandmother, who is helping to raise her two children (ages 1 month and 2 years). Hope does not go home every night, especially when she has been able to get high on her drug of choice, methamphetamine. She is worried she will be prosecuted for drug use or possession, and has been "laying low" to avoid being caught. One night after getting high, Hope is walking home alone and runs into her ex-boyfriend. They engage in a heated argument because her ex-boyfriend believes she has cash on her. He stabs her in the arm, a superficial wound, but with steady blood loss. She is rushed to the emergency department, where the wound is irrigated and sutured. The physician decides to ask for a psychiatric consult after assessing for symptoms of methamphetamine use.

APN Next Steps

Kailee is a PMHNP who performs consultation and liaison for the psychiatric department at the hospital. She is seeing Hope for her substance use disorder. During the consultation, the APN provides time for Hope to discuss the negative consequences of her methamphetamine use in her life. Hope describes her multigenerational home and her two young children. Kailee has been trained in motivational interviewing and uses these concepts to provide space for Hope to examine her life and set her goals, yet remaining nonjudgmental, offering empathy, and supporting self-efficacy. Kailee assesses Hope for any suicidal or violent thoughts or intentions. When these are negative, she offers Hope resources for an intensive outpatient program, at the community mental health clinic, which will provide

Hope with group therapy several days per week to assist in her road to recovery. Kailee understands how powerful addiction can be and that Hope has to decide for herself whether she is ready to take on this disease and live her life free from methamphetamine.

In view of the known substance use and chaos surrounding Hope's life currently, a report is called into the DCS, providing known information. Kailee understands that when there is suspected child abuse or neglect, it is the law that she report it.

□ □ □ □

Case Study 3: Mitchell

Mitchell, or Mitch, is a 45-year-old father diagnosed 3 months ago with stage IV lung cancer with bone metastasis. A heavy smoker, Mitch had not been to a health care provider for several years when his persistent cough, chronic fatigue, and loss of balance finally convinced him that he needed to be "checked out." Five years ago, his first wife divorced him, remarried, immediately started a new family (was pregnant when she divorced Mitch by the man she then married). At the time the divorce was finalized, she relinquished custody and terminated parental rights of their 4-year-old daughter. Mitch had done the best he could with an active daughter, Tanya, who is now 9 years of age.

The A-GNP, Maureen, who is also a hospice nurse, counsels Mitch as he makes arrangements for the parenting of his daughter. His ex-wife has requested the girl's aunt and uncle, her mother's sister and husband, care for the girl: "the only people I will allow to take my daughter," according to the birth mother. Mitch does not know them very well and has disregarded this request. During his divorce, his attorney advised him to draft a will stating that, in case of his passing, his parents would raise the child. Maureen also works with social services in obtaining a copy of Mitch's will. She speaks with the caseworker and emphasizes that Tanya will need grief counseling/individual counseling.

Four weeks later, it is apparent that the last round of chemotherapy has left Mitch weak, fatigued, and with severe thrombocytopenia. His immune system is not able to effectively fight infections, and he is admitted to the intensive care unit with sepsis, following a urinary tract infection. His laboratory results indicate multisystem organ failure, and he has requested to return home to die.

APN Next Steps

Mitch is transferred home, and continuous nursing care is initiated with orders for aggressive pain control and antinausea medication. All other medications are stopped. He becomes unresponsive with shallow breaths. Maureen verifies with nonverbal signs that he is comfortable, and checks his medical records that guardianship has been transferred to Mitch's parents. She sits next to Mitch's mother, sometimes in silence and taking her cues from the family in supportive care. She assures Mitch's mother that he is in no pain and that everything that can be done to fight his disease has been done.

She again emphasizes that Tanya and they will need emotional support after Mitch's passing and that she will assist in these referrals. She gently inquires whether social services has given her some options for counseling. His mother relates she was given information and a handout on children's grief reaction. As the family encircles his bed, Maureen hears Mitch's mother whisper in his ear a promise to "look after and protect Tanya." The next day, Mitch passes peacefully in his sleep.

□ □ □ □

CASE STUDY 4: HOLLY

Holly is 23 years old and has two biracial children by two different fathers. Each of the children was an "accident" from having unprotected sex. Both fathers are no longer in the environment and have little to do with Holly or the children. She lives at home with her mother, Kim, who is helping to raise her 2- and 4-year-old girls. Holly's father left the household when she was in second grade, and she has not heard from him since then. Kim works the evening shift as a respiratory therapy technician, and Holly works days as a store clerk at a gas station/pantry store. Together, they avoid childcare expenses and pool their money to make ends meet. Kim fixes the meals, and is the primary caretaker for the small girls and Holly.

Holly was diagnosed with asthma when she was 10 years old and relies on both controller (inhaled corticosteroids) and quick relief inhalers to keep her symptoms under control; however, she has missed her last two follow-up appointments with her provider. Unfortunately, Holly hates the side effects from the corticosteroids and is often nonadherent with the medication. Neither Kim nor Holly is a tobacco or drug user. Holly's typical symptoms include intermittent wheezing and coughing, and her sleep is often fitful. Every spring, Holly usually ends up in the emergency department for respiratory rescue because of the pollen and allergens in the air.

Holly is almost ready to take her General Education Development (GED) examination and hopes this will make her eligible for a promotion. After Kim arrives home from work, Holly will often go out with friends and sometimes does not come home. The children see Kim as their parent, whereas Holly is seen as more of an older sibling, although Kim insists that they call her "Grandma Kim." Kim has noticed that Holly has been having trouble sleeping and has complained about migraine headaches. Yesterday, she and Holly had a bitter fight after Holly stayed out all night, with Kim yelling, "These are your kids, not mine. If you get pregnant again, you can bet I'm not taking care of anymore of your kids!"

After work the following afternoon, Holly is in respiratory distress. Kim calls in sick to work, takes the children to a neighbor's house, and then transports Holly to an urgent care center, one that is familiar with Holly and her history with asthma.

APN Next Steps

Kristen, the primary care family nurse practitioner (FNP), is on staff at an urgent care center, an affiliate of the local acute care facility. She has seen Holly before, but is concerned today with her acute distress, current oxygen saturation of 91%, use of accessory muscles with respirations, lack of adherence to her treatment plan, and consistent use of the urgent care as her primary care provider.

Holly's initial assessment includes vital signs, general appearance, and focused assessment to include head, eye, ear, nose, mouth, throat, neck, respiratory, and cardiac systems. Holly is found to have wheezing in her lower respiratory tract with a prolonged expiratory phase. Initially, Holly is treated with ipratropium bromide (anticholinergic agent) in combination with albuterol (a short-acting beta-agonist) to provide quick relief of acute symptoms in the office. Holly is also placed on 2 L of oxygen. Once her oxygen saturations have reached 97% to 99% consistently and the use of accessory muscles has decreased, Holly is taken for a chest x-ray to rule out any differential diagnoses complicating cardiopulmonary processes. In addition, routine blood work is performed to include a complete blood count and a basic metabolic panel to assess for signs of infection, anemia, electrolyte imbalances, or kidney disease. The results of the chest x-ray and blood tests return as "negative," which allows for the definitive diagnosis of asthma exacerbation.

To treat Holly's current diagnosis, she is prescribed prednisolone 1 mg/kg/day for 7 days (systemic corticosteroids), budesonide inhaler, 360 mcg 1 puff twice daily (an inhaled corticosteroid as a long-term controller therapy), and albuterol MDI 2 puffs every 4 hours × 7 days and PRN thereafter. Kristen spends a considerable amount of time explaining to Holly the description and pathophysiology of asthma regarding its chronic nature, but ability to reverse the inflammatory airway disease with proper medication usage and regular follow-up. Risk factors such as allergens (environmental, medication, and food), tobacco smoke, lack of exercise, obesity, and increased stress were discussed. Kristen also explains the importance of following up with the allergist to which Holly is being referred. This provider will delve deeper into Holly's history and likely do allergy skin testing and breathing tests (spirometry and peak expiratory flow rates) in the office to determine the severity of Holly's asthma. In addition, this provider will develop an asthma treatment plan with Holly in consideration of her lifestyle, financial ability, and adherence, and continue to monitor and follow Holly's symptoms and health until her asthma is well controlled, hopefully reducing the number of times she is treated in urgent care or the emergency department.

Kristen is called briefly out of the room and returns to find Holly and Kim arguing loudly. Raised voices are heard about the cost of the visit and how "sick and tired" Kim is to continually have to take care of her daughter who should be more responsible and taking care of her own children. Holly starts to cry and begins to wheeze more pronouncedly.

Kristen begins to understand that this is a kinship family with multiple generations living in the same household. As Kristen is informed in the dynamics of kinship families, she uses techniques to de-escalate the situation.

"Your family is experiencing multiple stressors right now. The priority today is to help Holly control her asthma so that she can breathe easier."

Kim states, "I realize that. I'm just very tired." She glares at Holly, then softens. "I love my daughter, but there's nothing left for me—I never feel as if there is any time or energy left at the end of the day. I had to call off on *my* job today, something that I'll have to keep in mind whenever I'm feeling sick and want to call in. I'm constantly having to be the 'responsible' one, while she goes out partying with friends. Maybe if she partied less and took care of herself and her kids a little better, she wouldn't have these episodes."

Holly looks down, but remains silent.

Kristen nods. "I understand there's a lot going on and you both need to explore how you feel about the situation you currently have. There is a community mental health center that offers payment on a sliding scale. I'm going to give you the name of a therapist who might be able to help your family sort through all these. The center also offers parenting classes that may be helpful to you, Holly, so that you feel more empowered as a mother."

Both women seem calmer, and Kristen hands both the prescriptions and the therapist contact information to Holly. Kim murmurs, "thank you," and they leave the clinic.

APNs' Care of the Kinship Birth Parent

Kinship birth parents, although highly stigmatized, are at significant risk for substance use disorders, incarceration, and loss of their parental rights. Often seen as individuals who are creating trauma, they, themselves, may have experienced maltreatment. When we approach kinship birth parents, the interaction is as much about our attitudes as it is about knowledge and skills. If there has been maltreatment or substance use, APNs will need to fully grasp trauma-informed care and extend their perspective to include what the kinship birth parents have endured across their life span. The goal of reunification after incarceration or substance abuse treatment will also require an informed APN to collaborate with team members to decide what is in the best interest of the child (Table 7.1).

TABLE 7.1   *Kinship Birth Parents: What to Look for and What to Do*

Kinship Birth Parents

What to Look for (Assessment):

☐ Assess for substance use disorders, and for anxiety and depression in parents.
☐ Be alert for signs of child maltreatment.
☐ Assess coparenting with kinship caregiver, and monitor for solidarity in parenting.
☐ Assess for infectious diseases that are related to substance abuse disorders such as hepatitis C virus (HCV) and HIV.
☐ Assess for past trauma, using the ACE (adverse childhood experiences) index based on history of adverse experiences.

What to Do (Management):

☐ Report suspected or confirmed child maltreatment.
☐ Refer to social workers to optimize financial and social support as appropriate.
☐ Refer to substance abuse treatment programs, including intensive outpatient and residential rehabilitation.
☐ Refer to individual and family therapy as warranted.
☐ Encourage connecting with Narcotics Anonymous, Nar-Anon, Alcoholics Anonymous, and Al-Anon as indicated.
☐ Consult with experts in substance use disorders as needed.

CHAPTER HIGHLIGHTS

☐ Birth parents' involvement in the kinship household is along a continuum, from absence to coparenting.

☐ 2.3% of all children in the United States under 18 years have parents who are incarcerated. Substance abuse accounts for the majority of cases in which mothers are incarcerated and children are in foster care. Grandmothers are most frequently used to care for children of incarcerated mothers.

☐ The level of contact among kinship parents, children, and birth parents varies based on factors such as the level of child welfare involvement, substance use and mental health issues, and safety considerations.

☐ Few parents complete substance use treatment programs; however, those programs that coordinate services and bring services to the parents have demonstrated success in increasing these numbers.

☐ The medical and health care communities object to prosecution of pregnant women who are abusing substances. APNs have opportunities to offer management in a professional, nonjudgmental manner.

Questions for Reflection

Following are a few questions to reflect upon. You can use these to start a journal for yourself or in a classroom discussion with peers and the instructor.

1. What are your attitudes toward women who have involuntarily lost parental rights and have abused or neglected their children?
2. Should the federal government step forward and pass legislation that uniformly addresses how health care practitioners should report/treat expectant mothers/mothers who are abusing alcohol and/or drugs?
3. What issues of gender, race, and socioeconomic status do you think of when you address birth parents who are part of a kinship family?
4. Do you see birth parents as victims or criminals? If a substance abuser also has the diagnoses of posttraumatic stress disorder, depression, and is the victim of domestic violence, how does that change your narrative surrounding these patients? Families?
5. Which case study spoke to you the most? Why? What personal and professional feelings did it evoke within you?

References

Abrahams, R., Albizu-Garcia, C., Bakker, A., Behnke, M., Cambell, N., Chasnoff, I. J., . . . Zobin, M. (2013, March 11). Open letter to the media and policy makers regarding alarmist and inaccurate reporting on prescription opioid use by pregnant women. Retrieved from advocatesforpregnantwomen.org/Opioid%20Open%20Letter%20-%20 March%202013%20-%20FINAL.pdf

Child Welfare Information Gateway. (2011). *About CAPTA: A legislative history*. Washington, DC: U.S. Department of Health and Human Services, Children's Bureau.

Child Welfare Information Gateway. (2016). *Mandatory reporters of child abuse and neglect.* Washington, DC: U.S. Department of Health and Human Services, Children's Bureau.

Conn, A. M., Szilagyi, M. A., Franke, T. M., Albertin, C. S., Blumkin, A. K., & Szilagyi, P. G. (2013). Trends in child protection and out-of-home care. *Pediatrics, 132*(4), 712–719. doi:10.1542/peds.2013–0969

Glaze, L. E., & Maruschak, L. M. (2010). *Special report: Parents in prison and their minor children.* Washington, DC: U.S. Department of Justice, Bureau of Justice Statistics. Retrieved from www.bjs.gov/content/pub/pdf/pptmc.pdf

Green, Y. R., & Goodman, C. C. (2010). Understanding birth parent involvement in kinship families: Influencing factors and the importance of placement arrangement. *Children and Youth Services Review, 32,* 1357–1364. doi:10.1016/j.childyouth.2010.06.003

Haight, W. L., Carter-Black, J. D., & Sheridan, K. (2009). Mothers' experience of methamphetamine addiction: A case-based analysis of rural, midwestern women. *Children and Youth Services Review, 31,* 71–77. doi:10.1016/j.childyouth.2008.05.011

Narcotics Anonymous. (2006/2014). Information about NA. Retrieved from na.org/admin/include/spaw2/uploads/pdf/PR/Information_about_NA.pdf

Oliveros, A., & Kaufman, J. (2011). Addressing substance abuse treatment needs of parents involved with the child welfare system. *Child Welfare, 90*(1), 25–41.

The Sentencing Project. (2007). *Women in the criminal justice system: Briefing sheets.* Washington, DC: Author. Retrieved from http://www.sentencingproject.org/wp-content/uploads/2016/01/Women-in-the-Criminal-Justice-System-Briefing-Sheets.pdf

Smith, A., Krisman, K., Strozier, A., & Marley, M. (2004). Breaking through the bars: Exploring the experience of addicted incarcerated parents whose children are cared for by relatives. *Families in Society: The Journal of Contemporary Social Services, 85*(2), 187–195.

Strozier, A., Armstrong, M., Skuza, S, Cecil, D., & McHale, J. (2011). Coparenting in kinship families with incarcerated mothers: A qualitative study. *Families in Society: The Journal of Contemporary Social Services, 92*(1), 55–61. doi:10.1606/1044-3894.4064

Traube, D. E., He, A. S., Zhu, L., Scalise, C., & Richardson, T. (2015). Predictors of substance abuse assessment and treatment completion for parents involved with child welfare: One state's experience in matching across systems. *Child Welfare, 94*(5), 45–66.

University of California, San Francisco. (2016). Clinical consultation center. Retrieved from http://nccc.ucsf.edu/clinician-consultation /substance-use-management

Young, N. K., Boles, S. M., & Otero, C. (2007). Parental substance use disorders and child maltreatment: Overlap, gaps, and opportunities. *Child Maltreatment, 12*, 137–149. doi:10.1177/1077559507300322

8

Kinship Children

□ □ □ □

PURPOSE OF THE CHAPTER

Children under the care of kin have transitioned from at least one home prior to their placement in the kinship caregiver's home. As with the population of children who are removed to reside with nonrelative foster parents, these children have often experienced maltreatment and traumatic events. Children adopted by relatives have experienced more emotional trauma, neglect, and for children younger than 6 years of age, more physical abuse than children adopted by nonrelatives (Foli, Lim, & Sands, 2015). Yet, despite these histories, overall, the evidence supports better outcomes for children who are placed with kin, especially older children (Wu, White, & Coleman, 2015).

We discuss four kinship care cases that highlight the twists and turns of kinship care: a young girl who is in the care of her aunt; a 10-year-old boy who is being raised by his grandmother; a teenage girl who dreams of traveling across the country to be reunited with her birth mother; and a newborn with neonatal abstinence syndrome (NAS) who is discharged into the care of her older sibling.

Learning Objectives

At the completion of the chapter, the reader will be able to:

1. Understand that the surge of children formally placed with relatives through the foster care system accounts for only a portion of this growing population
2. Differentiate the outcomes for children placed with relatives/kin from those for children placed with nonrelatives/kin
3. Review the health disparities faced by children in kinship care

IMPACT OF KINSHIP CARE ON CHILDREN

As previously outlined, the Fostering Connections to Success and Increasing Adoptions Act of 2008 requires caseworkers to attempt to locate relatives within 30 days of removal from the birth parent home; this has resulted in a surge of relative placements of children in the foster care system. As of July 2015, the Adoption and Foster Care Analysis Reporting System (AFCARS, 2015) reveals how widespread kinship placement is in the foster care system. Twenty-nine percent, or more than 120,000 children, are living in relative foster care placements. Interestingly, in 2014, almost one third of adoptions (32%) with public agency involvement were by relatives (AFCARS, 2015). However, these figures *do not include* children who are not in the child welfare system.

The figures from the Current Population Survey Annual Social and Economic Supplement (Kids Count Data Center, 2015) tell us the story about kinship children who are not in foster care placement (working with child welfare). For the period 2013 through 2015, 3% of all children (2.5 million) in the United States resided in kinship families, with the highest percentage in West Virginia (7%) and the lowest in Utah, Wisconsin, Oregon, Minnesota, Iowa, Maine, Michigan, Nebraska, New Jersey, Illinois, and Iowa, at 2% each. It is important to note that these figures reflect when "the child is not a foster child to the householder." Therefore, it would seem these figures *do not include* those children in the care of relatives who are in the foster care system (Kids Count Data Center, 2015).

What are the outcomes for children cared for by kinship parents? In a systematic review of 62 quasi-experimental studies that compared kinship and foster care outcomes for children, Winokur, Holtan, and Valentine (2009) concluded the following:

> . . . it appears that children in kinship care experience better outcomes in regard to behavior problems, adaptive behaviors, psychiatric disorders, well-being, placement stability, and guardianship than do children in foster care. (p. 34)

However, a frequent theme in kinship care is that mental health services are less likely to be used than for children in nonkinship out of home care (Winokur, Holtan, & Valentine, 2009). When matched demographically with children in foster care, kinship children are also less likely to be involved in the juvenile justice system, have fewer placements, allegations of new abuse and neglect, and achieve reunification (Winokur, Crawford, Longobardi, & Valentine, 2008). Unfortunately, one caveat to all of this evidence is that most, if not all, has been collected from kinship families who are also in the child welfare/foster care system. The outcomes for families that are "off the grid" are very difficult to capture.

PLACEMENT AND PERMANENCY

There are also outcomes that address ties with siblings—indeed, a family network—as well as a sense of culture and identity that children benefit from when in kinship care (Kiraly & Humphreys, 2013). Children in kinship care more often have the ability to access information and to have a sense of "why" they are where they are. Still, others argue that placement of children in kinship care often lacks close evaluation. Factors such as the age and health of the kinship caregiver, the safety of the contact with birth parents who may experience substance use disorders and mental health issues, and other less straightforward parameters may be overlooked as placements are considered.

Benefits to older children, ages 6 to 17.5 years, have been found when compared with nonkinship care placement. These benefits included lower internalizing, externalizing, and total behavioral problems (Wu et al., 2015). However, the benefits to younger children were less clear and not statistically significant when compared with nonkinship care (Wu et al., 2015). Koh (2010) reported findings from matched kinship and nonkinship families across five states using AFCARS data. States varied by White and African American kinship parent mix, with some states having equal numbers of racial backgrounds (Connecticut and Tennessee), more White kinship families (Arizona), and more African American (Missouri and Ohio). Across states, kinship parents were likely to be older and single, with kinship arrangements showing advantages to permanency placements, defined as guardianship and adoption. Koh (2010) also identified state-by-state differences in how kinship families were integrated into the foster care system as worthy of further exploration.

Children living with kin are a growing phenomenon across English-speaking countries, (e.g., England and Australia), and generalizability of research findings conducted by these countries should be noted. Research indicates, overall, the positive benefits of kinship care, with protective factors such as the closeness of relationship and placement stability, which can offset poorer environmental conditions and poorer quality of care (Brown & Sen, 2014). Kin placements that are not in the best interest of the child, however, should be considered, despite the children's preference for its continuance (Brown & Sen, 2014). A qualitative study of 80 children living in informal kinship arrangements in England found strong attachment to their caregivers, but also feeling stigmatized by their living arrangement (Farmer, Selwyn, & Meakings, 2013). Anecdotally, I can confirm the study results. During the class that I teach for kinship parents, many kinship parents have voiced how important it is for their children to be able to interact with other children in similar situations. They wished that the schools the children attended would host support groups for kinship children. Two children discovered during one class that they attended the same school, but were unaware the other was also living with grandparents.

In a mixed methods study of 694 kinship families conducted in Australia, Kiraly and Humphreys (2016) describe children's contact with parents and others. One significant finding was that 204 or 39% of the kinship providers reported that during visits with birth mothers, "children's safety had been compromised" (p. 232); the other half of the sample reported positive experiences. The wide network of kinship arrangements, including contacts with siblings and extended family, were viewed as benefits (Kiraly & Humphreys, 2016). The issue of safety was echoed (during the trauma-informed classes) by kinship providers who reported to me that they now insist on supervised visits in public places, "because they [birth parents] seem to act better in public." Other kinship providers describe how the children have significant externalizing behaviors (i.e., spitting in the birth parent's face) when their birth parent is in the environment, and the subsequent chaos that would erupt during and after visits.

The evidence offers us preliminary glimpses of how kinship arrangements may afford the child more stability, permanency arrangements, and psychological buffers. However, the gaps in the literature are also apparent. With kinship parent demographics creating at-risk profiles (single parents, older, more likely to be below the poverty level, and chronic health difficulties), the health outcomes of children in kinship placements remain relatively unexplored. As kinship children may not be in contact with the child welfare system, these questions increase in importance. Washington, Gleeson, and Rulison (2013) examined African American kinship families who had an informal arrangement (not involved in the child welfare system) and considered the child outcome of competence. The average scores of the quality of the relationship between the birth mother and birth father and the child in kinship care and the average scores of child competency were positively associated. Other positive relationships with child competence include healthier kinship family functioning and caregiver social support (Washington, Gleeson, & Rulison, 2013).

Future research should examine factors that relate to mental health functioning for children and adolescents in kinship families, such as gender, parental history of mental health problems, placement stability, relationships with adults, school services, safety/lack of maltreatment while in care, history of sexual abuse, and leaving care (running away) (Fechter-Leggett & O'Brien, 2010). Health outcomes should also be explored, including those indicated by adverse childhood experiences (ACEs).

CASE STUDIES: KINSHIP CHILDREN

□ □ □ □

CASE STUDY 1: TAYLOR

Taylor is a 5-year-old girl who attends regular classes at a public elementary school. She presents to her pediatric nurse practitioner (PNP) for a well-child check and review of immunizations accompanied by her aunt, Kathy, who is raising Taylor. She became a kinship parent when her sister remarried and wanted to begin a new family with her husband; they have since relocated out of state. Kathy, a 42-year-old small business owner of a women's boutique, has flexible hours. She had always wanted to be a mother and felt that the "stars had aligned." Taylor was always a bit odd and one of those children who tended to be bullied and left out. Something in Kathy wanted to help Taylor and knew that her sister's new husband did not seem able to bond with the child. Kathy agreed to take Taylor and raise her as her own child, insisting on legal guardianship.

Although Kathy has been caring for Taylor only for a few months, Taylor's teachers are increasingly concerned with her inability to stay with her peers academically. Kathy has noticed behavioral problems as well, because Taylor does not seem to listen and asks her to repeat directions, saying "What?" many times. Taylor is unorganized and her room is messy, despite Kathy's attempts to help her straighten it. Taylor's teacher also reports disruptive behaviors in class, taking crayons away from others without asking, and putting on other students' coats.

Bonnie, the PNP, asks Kathy for a health history, which seems unremarkable as all developmental milestones have been met. Bonnie reviews the immunization chart and recognizes that Taylor needs the fifth dose of diphtheria, tetanus, and acellular pertussis (DTaP); the fourth dose of the inactivated poliovirus (IPV); the second dose of measles, mumps, and rubella (MMR); and the second dose of the varicella (VAR) vaccines.

Bonnie then asks Kathy about information related to her sister's pregnancy and whether there were any complications. Kathy hesitates and then relates that her sister drank intermittently during the pregnancy. Hurrying to her sister's defense, she tells Bonnie how stressful it had been for her sister. At the time she was pregnant, she was also divorcing her first husband. Kathy relates that she is just not sure how much alcohol her sister consumed, stating: "She called me several times, clearly drunk. I didn't know how to help her. . . ."

APN Next Steps

Bonnie begins to suspect fetal alcohol spectrum disorders (FASDs) with the potential for alcohol-related neurodevelopmental disorder (ARND). She performs a physical examination on Taylor and is uncertain whether the facial signs of FASD are evident (smooth ridge between nose and upper lip). She notes that Taylor is in the lower 10th percentile in the growth chart for both height and weight. Recognizing the potential for the learning differences and behavior issues reported by Kathy, Bonnie refers Taylor to a developmental pediatrician to conduct further testing, including in the area of FASD.

Kathy becomes upset and states, "Oh no, no, no. I can't handle this."

Bonnie sits down beside Kathy and asks the medical assistant to play with Taylor in the waiting area. Bonnie explains what FASD is and that there are a range of symptoms and issues when a child is born to a person who has consumed alcohol during the pregnancy. Her eyes brimming with tears, Kathy blurts out, "It figures. My sister screwed up. And once again, I'm left holding the bag."

Bonnie offers therapeutic silence for a few seconds. Kathy finally says in a small voice, "I'm sorry. I love my sister, and I love Taylor. I'll do what it takes to ensure Taylor's okay."

Bonnie responds that she understands how this news must be overwhelming, and commends Kathy on her commitment to Taylor's well-being. She also cautions Kathy that until Taylor is evaluated by a specialist, she should not conclude anything about Taylor's diagnosis.

Follow-Up

Four months later, Bonnie sees Taylor for complaints of a sore throat. After examining Taylor, Bonnie assures Kathy the symptoms indicate a viral infection and recommends treatment with fluids and acetaminophen for pain. Kathy then relates that the developmental pediatrician's examination is consistent with the diagnosis of fetal alcohol syndrome (FAS) in all areas: three abnormal facial features, growth problems, central nervous system deficits, and a history of alcohol use by the mother while pregnant. Recommendations are to follow up in the FAS clinic in 1 month to implement an individualized treatment plan.

Kathy admits she is having trouble not blaming her sister for all this "heartache" and "hurting Taylor like she did." Bonnie listens patiently, advising Kathy to consider counseling for herself to process her anger and follow up with her primary care provider as needed.

CASE STUDY 2: JARRED

A 10-year-old boy, Jarred, is being seen by a psychiatric mental health nurse practitioner (PMHNP), Barb, for follow-up on medication to manage his attention deficit hyperactivity disorder (ADHD). He is accompanied by his 62-year-old grandmother, Margaret, his kinship parent. While Jarred waits outside the room, Margaret reports that although Jarred seems to be able to concentrate more and is less "hyper," he has begun to be oppositional and "melts down" when he does not get his own way. She recently has required the children to attend Sunday church services with her. His teachers report that he is able to attend better in class. However, they also report that his emotions swing widely, and he has been verbally aggressive to his peers, which is a new behavior for him. At home, Margaret reports similar issues, especially when Jarred is tired or at bedtime. He pushed his 5-year-old sister, whom she is also raising, last night, creating chaos in the home. Margaret asked why Jarred would do that, and he replied that his sister would not do what he had told her to do.

Margaret has instituted a system of rewards and knows that Jarred enjoys playing videogames. A game he has been wanting for months is about ready to be released, and he is close to earning enough "good behavior points" to buy it. But Margaret feels these new behaviors should not be rewarded and is reconsidering allowing the purchase.

Barb listens closely and has reviewed Jarred's records. He came to Margaret's care when he was 7 years old and has been on methylphenidate sustained release for approximately 6 months. Initially, reports pointed to substantial improvement in Jarred's behaviors. The school, working with Margaret, had instituted an individual education plan for Jarred, who was considered above normal intelligence. So far, he is not in any special education programs.

APN Next Steps

While Margaret waits in the patient lounge area, Barb begins her focused assessment with Jarred, asking what he enjoys doing the most. His face brightens, and he describes the upcoming game he will be buying because "I've been so good." Barb continues to discuss the game and weaves into the assessment questions about how he felt when he took his pill, and asks specific questions about common side effects and how his appetite is. His weight is stable, and he has gained 2 pounds since his last visit 3 months ago. Then, Barb asks about his sister and how she is doing. Jarred becomes quiet and will not answer.

Barb reflects this behavior: "You became quiet, Jarred." The boy begins describing how his "feelings overflow." He becomes tearful and blurts out, "What happened to my parents? They were mean to me. Did they go to hell? Am I going to hell?"

Barb begins to understand that Jarred has experienced traumatic events; coupled with attending church services and having his ADHD symptoms under control, his traumatic stress has surfaced. She understands that the goals of children who have experienced trauma are to feel safe and in control of the environment. She knows, depending on the trauma's duration and severity, Jarred's brain development was affected. What could easily have been attributed to his ADHD, was in actuality, related to his inability to control and cope with residual fear from a history of maltreatment and traumatic events.

In the ensuing weeks, Barb continues to peel off the layers of trauma in one-on-one therapy with Jarred. She also educates Margaret on trauma's effects on children, emphasizing that when the trauma occurred in his development is also important.

Jarred is able to buy his game as promised, and Margaret is able to interpret Jarred's behaviors in a trauma-informed way. When needed, she redirects Jarred, but also continues to assure him that he is safe and gives him choices as much as she can. As Jarred seeks ways to control his environment and those around him, Margaret and his teacher work together to ensure boundaries and rules are clear so he feels safe, and those around him feel safe.

□ □ □ □

CASE STUDY 3: LINDSEY

Lindsey is 16 years old, and her main aspiration in life is to get a driver's license and leave her grandmother's home, where she has been living for the past 5 years. She longs to reconnect with her birth mother, and does not understand why she and her two brothers cannot live as a family with their mother. Her grandmother, Raya, is too strict, enforcing a curfew and taking away privileges if she does not make at least Bs in her classes at school. And Raya is too old to understand what Lindsey is going through. She does not fit in at school and never will. All Lindsey wants to do is run away. Each time she tries to ask Raya about her mother, Raya firmly says she does not want to talk about her.

Lindsey never knew her dad, and her brothers are actually half-siblings whose father has since divorced her mom. The last time she heard from her mom, Cindi, was last fall—a postcard from

Texas, saying she missed Lindsey. Now, having turned 16, it is time to put her plan into action.

Before she can leave, Raya has an appointment set up for Lindsey to be rechecked for anemia. Her menses is very heavy and these symptoms are getting worse, including significant cramping with each period. The PNP is considering prescribing birth control pills so that her periods will be lighter. Lindsey hopes that she does—she would like to meet someone and does not want to get pregnant as her mother did when she was 16.

Raya takes Lindsey to the community health center, which is a federally qualified health center (FQHC) primarily staffed by nurse practitioners. Raya pays on a sliding scale for health care services for herself and her grandchildren. Mary, the PNP, sees Lindsey for her appointment. This is Lindsey's third appointment with Mary, who is aware of her kinship status. Lindsey has a history of physical abuse by her mother's boyfriends and significant emotional and physical neglect before she began living with Raya 5 years ago.

APN Next Steps

Raya sits with Lindsey while Mary reviews the complete blood count findings; her hemoglobin is 10.8 g/dL, indicating that she has iron-deficiency anemia. Mary takes an updated history of Lindsey's periods: frequency, duration, intensity and decides to prescribe oral contraceptives. Raya steps out while Mary does a brief physical exam on Lindsey.

Mary notices that Lindsey appears very happy to learn of the prescription, and she decides to ask follow-up questions. She asks Lindsey what she enjoys doing the most, and Lindsey replies that she is looking forward to driving. Mary continues to probe and realizes that Lindsey has plans to "travel on her own" and that if she takes "the pill," she "cannot get pregnant, right?"

Mary advises that the medication will not protect her against sexually transmitted infections. She is concerned about Lindsey and asks her if she is planning to take Raya and her brothers on the trip. Lindsey becomes quiet and sullen. Mary pauses in the physical exam and looks at Lindsey. Because Mary is adoption/kinship-informed, she know this conversation is important and how to begin: "Lindsey, it sounds as if you've made some pretty definite plans."

Lindsey hesitates, but states, "Yeah. I guess so."

"It must be difficult at times, trying to understand all that's happened to you."

Lindsey looks down and blinks, trying to hold back tears. "I guess," she whispers.

"What are your questions? Maybe I can help answer some of them."

Lindsey then asks why her mother cannot take care of her and her brothers. She is convinced that if she can make contact with her mother, she will let Lindsey live with her again. She tells Mary about the postcard. Mary listens and nods, summarizing and restating what Lindsey tells her.

Finally, Mary says, "Lindsey, are you planning to try to find your mother without telling your grandmother?"

Lindsey nods and begins to cry. Mary feels an ethical dilemma: should she tell the grandmother, Raya, about Lindsey's plans? What is Mary's liability if Lindsey runs away without telling Raya, and Lindsey is harmed? What about patient confidentiality? Should Mary respect Lindsey's confidence and handle the situation without involving Raya?

After deliberation, Mary understands that Lindsey is running toward her mother, not necessarily away from Raya, her grandmother. She appreciates all of the questions and unknown pieces to Lindsey's life. Mary knows it is important for Lindsey to talk with her grandmother and shares, "I wonder if your grandmother knows how important it is for you to know more about your mother." Mary asks Lindsey to bring Raya into the office and share her feelings, saying, "I can see how painful this is for you, and it's important that your grandmother understand your feelings also."

Mary gently encourages Lindsey to explain to Raya about how important it is for Lindsey to know more about her past and what has happened to her mother. She also educates Lindsey on how dangerous it would be for her to embark on a trip to find her mother by herself. She asks Lindsey about why Raya may be hesitant to talk about Lindsey's mother, Cindi. It may be because of hurt, guilt, shame, worry, and helplessness—or even an attempt to protect Lindsey. She should not assume it is because she does not want Lindsey to know her mother.

Lindsey agrees to have Mary bring Raya into the room and promises not to run away, but insists that when she is 18, she will, if she has to. After Raya is settled, Mary asks Lindsey to convey that she would like to try to find Cindi. Raya begins to react, but catches herself when Mary rests her hand on her arm. Mary knows she is running late for her next appointment, and summarizes what has transpired and her recommendations: Physical management of iron-deficiency anemia related to heavy menses; recheck iron levels in 3 months; prescription for slow-release iron and birth control pills; psychosocial management: refer to psychiatric mental health nurse practitioner for individual and family therapy at the clinic (the PMHNP is at the clinic 2 days/week). Last, Mary encourages Raya and Lindsey to keep communicating, remembering the rules of respect and turn-taking.

□ □ □ □

CASE STUDY 4: ABIGAIL

Abigail's mother, Wendy, has two families: four children whom she parented for 20 years with her ex-husband, and the pregnancy with Abigail with a partner she barely knew. Her first family lived in a rural Midwestern town, and when the factory that employed most of the population closed, money was tight. Abigail's mother and father started working two jobs to make ends meet for their four children, ages 13 to 20 years of age. Unfortunately, Abigail's mother, was influenced by some of her friends who encouraged her to try heroin as a stress reliever; she became addicted, and 1 year later, the couple divorced. Abigail's mother fell into a homeless state and became pregnant by an acquaintance. Wendy's first husband, the father to the four children, worked to provide stability for them, and when he learned "through the town grapevine" that his ex-wife was homeless and pregnant, he went looking for her. Despite protest from Wendy, he insisted she get prenatal care, and she was placed on a regimen of buprenorphine, a partial mu-opioid agonist, used for opioid-dependent pregnant women.

Three months later, Abigail was born. After 24 hours, Wendy left the hospital and gave guardianship to her oldest daughter, Erin. Because of respiratory depression, Abigail was placed in the neonatal intensive care unit (NICU) and was closely monitored for neonatal abstinence syndrome (NAS). Because Abigail's mother received buprenorphine, her NAS symptoms were manageable: mild diarrhea and a high-pitched cry that abated with comfort. Abigail's oldest half-sibling, Erin, just graduated from nursing school and intends to raise Abigail.

APN Next Steps

Anna is a PNP in a busy community health clinic. Her practice is overseen by a collaborating physician, whom she consults on a regular basis. Today, she is seeing a 2-week-old infant for a well-child exam who was discharged 4 days postdelivery with mild NAS symptoms. The mother, however, reports the baby girl has been sweating and has had some loose stools in the past 48 hours; but the baby's fluid intake is good, and she is sucking well from a bottle. Anna begins to ask about breastfeeding, when Erin stops her and says, "I'm her sister, so that's not an option. I'm a nurse, though, so that helps. I understand that Abigail has prenatal NAS."

Erin goes on to explain her situation and how she has assumed the care of Abigail, intending to someday adopt the child. Anna nods and listens closely. She then completes a newborn assessment on Abigail, with a special emphasis on central nervous system (CNS) functioning, autonomic dysfunction (such as tachypnea, sneezing, and excessive yawning), and gastrointestinal (GI) functioning (including regurgitation). She also notes that Abigail is at risk for skin breakdown and instructs Erin on preventive measures as well as other nonpharmacological interventions (see Table 8.1; MacMullen, Dulski, & Blobaum, 2014).

Anna is overall reassured that Abigail's physical and neurological exam indicates that nursing and comfort measures will be enough to allow her body to rebound from the NAS. Anna spends time, however, ensuring Erin understands how important these measures are. She explains how Abigail's body is adapting to living without the drug that her mother received. Anna also notes the bonding between the mother and daughter. Erin maintains eye contact with Abigail, who also reacts to Erin's voice, which is soothing as she swaddles the baby and gently picks her up, supporting Abigail's head. Anna provides anticipatory guidance on signs and symptoms that may indicate a need for more aggressive treatment (e.g., continuation or worsening of GI upset, fever, increased sweating, and seizures) that warrant Erin's contacting the clinic immediately.

TABLE 8.1   *Evidence-based Nursing Interventions for Infants With Neonatal Abstinence Syndrome (NAS)*

- ☐ Do a thorough, accurate maternal history to determine whether the neonate will be at risk. A drug history is included for all pregnant women, not just those who are suspected or confirmed substance abusers.
- ☐ Screen all infants at risk with a reliable and valid NAS scoring instrument, which typically assesses symptoms of withdrawal and assigns a score in accordance with the severity of the symptoms.
- ☐ Provide supportive measures, such as swaddling, decreased stimulation, supine (or others as appropriate) positioning, massage, cuddling.
- ☐ Correct nutritional deficiencies with appropriate therapy (e.g., high-calorie formula, gavage feeds, IV therapy).
- ☐ Encourage the maternal–neonatal relationship through support for breastfeeding and rooming-in if there are no contraindications.
- ☐ Administer topical ointments or barrier shields for skin breakdown.
- ☐ Administer and monitor pharmacologic treatment if withdrawal is not contained by supportive measures. Gradually wean when appropriate.
- ☐ Collect samples for laboratory testing, if ordered.
- ☐ Assess and reassess NAS symptoms; if severe, act to prevent complications.
- ☐ Communicate and provide referral to a social worker or other personnel for follow-up postdischarge.
- ☐ Provide parenting education to caretakers of the neonate.
- ☐ Promote sleep by clustering interventions to avoid sleep disruption.

Source: MacMullen et al. (2014).

Follow-Up

Abigail is here for her well-child exam and follow-up visit 2 weeks later. The baby is more alert, grimacing less, and has gained 16 ounces. Erin smiles when she reports on Abigail's progress, including less crying, sleeping longer, and even smiling and cooing when spoken to. Anna's assessment of Abigail reveals a healthy 1-month-old who is growing and developing normally. CNS, autonomic, and GI symptoms are decreasing. Anna witnesses Erin's gentleness with the infant, engagement with the baby through soft coos, and ensuring the baby is wrapped in her blanket.

APNS' CARE OF KINSHIP CHILDREN

Vulnerable, at-risk, health disparities, chronic, complex trauma: Many of these adjectives aptly describe children in kinship families.

Their parents may be incarcerated, and their current caregivers are often older and have chronic health care needs of their own. In other words, their parentage may be absent or incapable of meeting their needs. Informed APNs can draw upon what they know about the benefits of kinship parenting and view the family system as a whole, supporting the competency of the kinship parent yet ensuring the child's needs are met. APNs will often be the first point of contact with these at-risk children, and collaborations with team members will be important (Table 8.2).

TABLE 8.2 *Kinship Children: What to Look for and What to Do*

Kinship Children

What to Look for (Assessment):

☐ Follow assessment guidelines as outlined in Chapter 2 and per the American Academy of Pediatrics.
☐ Assess adverse childhood experiences (ACE) indicators in children whose history indicates the potential for trauma.
☐ Monitor for signs of psychological distress, including depression, suicidal ideation/plans, and substance use disorders.
☐ Tease out physical complaints that may be related to psychosocial needs.
☐ Assess for microaggressions against being a member of a kinship family, which may include an incarcerated parent.
☐ Assess the relationship with birth parents, and kinship parents' social support to facilitate competency in the child.

What to Do (Management):

☐ Provide psychosocial support and therapeutic communication before and after placement with kinship.
☐ Support reunification efforts as appropriate.
☐ Refer children and adolescents to needed resources to strengthen health and their role in society.
☐ Provide continuity of medical and health care services for kinship children.
☐ Provide education to kinship parents regarding trauma behaviors such as food hoarding, externalizing (aggressive behaviors, acting out), and internalizing behaviors (depression, withdrawal from family/friends).
☐ Dialogue with kinship children/adolescents to facilitate feelings of safety, capability, and control.
☐ Report suspected or confirmed child abuse and neglect.

CHAPTER HIGHLIGHTS

☐ The number of children under the care of kinship parents is significantly increasing in the United States.

☐ Relative and kin placement is the first choice when children have been removed from their birth parents.

☐ Kinship children often have histories that are significant for maltreatment and trauma; behaviors stemming from these can be misattributed to other mental health issues.

☐ Systematic and literature reviews consistently report positive child welfare and psychological outcomes for children in kinship care when compared with children in nonrelative foster care.

☐ Not all kinship placements may be in the best interest of the child, and various factors should be weighed carefully by the health care team.

Questions for Reflection

Following are a few questions to reflect upon. You can use these to start a journal for yourself or in a classroom discussion with peers and the instructor.

1. How do you identify children and adolescents who are under the care of family and fictive kin? How do you incorporate this information into your management plan?

2. How do you incorporate developmental stages and trauma-informed care into your practice with kinship children and adolescents? Why are these layers of knowledge important with these vulnerable groups of patients?

3. How do you balance the needs of a child who may not be receiving adequate care by a kinship parent, but who may feel a significant attachment to them? How would you rate the following in importance to a child who has been maltreated by his/her birth parents: placement stability, environment, financial resources, and family connections?

4. When you consider kinship children, who are your collaborators? How does team science manifest itself in the care of this group?

5. Which case study spoke to you the most? Why? What personal and professional feelings did it evoke within you?

References

Adoption and Foster Care Analysis and Reporting System. (2015). Preliminary estimates for FY 2014 as of July 2015. *The AFCARS Report, 22,* 1–6.

Brown, L., & Sen, R. (2014). Improving outcomes for looked after children: A critical analysis of kinship care. *Practice: Social Work in Action, 26*(3), 161–180. doi:10.1080/09503153.2014. 914163

Farmer, E., Selwyn, J., & Meakings, S. (2013). "Other children say you're not normal because you don't live with your parents." Children's views of living with informal kinship carers: Social networks, stigma and attachment to carers. *Child and Family Social Work, 18,* 25–34. doi:10.1111 /cfs.12030

Fechter-Leggett, M. O., & O'Brien, K. (2010). The effects of kinship care on adult mental health outcomes of alumni of foster care. *Children and Youth Services Review, 32*(2), 206–213. doi:10.1016/j.childyouth.2009.08.017

Foli, K. J., Lim, E., & Sands, L. P. (2015). Comparison of relative and non-relative adoptive parent health status. *Western Journal of Nursing Research, 37*(3), 320–341. doi:10.1177/0193945913511708

Kids Count Data Center. (2015). Children in kinship care. Retrieved from datacenter.kidscount.org/data/tables/7172-children-in-kinship-care? loc=1&loct=2#ranking/1/any/true/1491/any/14207

Kiraly, M., & Humphreys, C. (2013). Family contact for children in kinship care: A literature review. *Australian Social Work, 66*(3), 358–374. doi:10.10 80/0312407X.2013.812129

Kiraly, M., & Humphreys, C. (2016). "It's about the whole family": Family contact for children in kinship care. *Child and Family Social Work, 21,* 228–239. doi:10.1111/cfs.12140

Koh, E. (2010). Permanency outcomes of children in kinship and non-kinship foster care: Testing the external validity of kinship effects. *Children and Youth Services, 32,* 389–398. doi:10.1016/j.childyouth.2009.10.010

MacMullen, N. J., Dulski, L. A., & Blobaum, P. (2014). Evidence-based interventions for neonatal abstinence syndrome. *Pediatric Nursing, 40*(4), 165–172, 203.

Washington, T., Gleeson, J. P., & Rulison, K. L. (2013). Competence and African American children in informal kinship care: The role of family. *Children and Youth Services, 35,* 1305–1312. doi:10.1016/jchildyouth.2013.05.011

Winokur, M. A., Crawford, G. A., Longobardi, R. C., & Valentine, D. P. (2008). Matched comparison of children in kinship care and foster care on child welfare outcomes. *Child Welfare and Foster Care, 89*(3), 338–346. doi:10.1606/1044-3894.3759

Winokur, M., Holtan, A., & Valentine, D. (2009). Kinship care for the safety, permanency, and well-being of children removed from the home for maltreatment. *Campbell Systematic Reviews, 1.* doi:10.4073/csr.2009.1

Wu, Q., White, K. R., & Coleman, K. L. (2015). Effects of kinship care on behavioral problems by child age: A propensity score analysis. *Children and Youth Services Review, 57,* 1–8.

9

Special Cases: Foster Care, Assisted Reproductive Technology, Commercial Surrogacy, and Human Trafficking

□ □ □ □

PURPOSE OF THE CHAPTER

This discussion is a collection of topics that relate to nontraditional families, but do not quite belong in the previous chapters. Nonetheless, the subjects are important to advanced practice nurses' (APNs') care delivery. Some of the issues are related to technological advances, and others to the debasement of human beings, which occurs in human trafficking. Still other areas covered in this chapter are devoted to the children in foster care who await permanent placement—fancy words for an adoptive family to love them and give them a home. Many of them will be reunited with their birth parents, whereas some will become part of an adoptive family or be placed with a relative/ kinship parent. But some will linger in the foster care system and eventually reach the age of emancipation or "aging out" of foster care. This chapter is devoted to these children and adolescents and the needs that can be met by APNs.

Learning Objectives

At the completion of the chapter, the reader will be able to:

1. Identify various situations that may emerge in foster care; for example, reunification with birth parents, multiple placements in foster homes, and legal adoption of children in foster care

2. Analyze select systems in the foster care system as they relate to medical needs and levels of care
3. Compare and contrast the dynamics of foster parenting with adoptive and kinship parenting
4. Describe the changes in adoption that are driven by technology, specifically, embryo donation and global commercial surrogacy
5. Discuss the Unaccompanied Refugee Minors program
6. Analyze the vulnerabilities of children in the foster care system as targets of human trafficking, especially those who "age out of the system"

FOSTER PARENTS AND CHILDREN

May is National Foster Care Month and recognizes those individuals who provide a home and family to children in the welfare system. *The Fosters*, a television show that was originally broadcast in June 2013, portrays a same-sex couple with birth, adopted, and foster children. It was one of the first television programs to depict a foster family. In contrast, the media has reported situations where foster parents have themselves been the perpetrators of maltreatment of children under their care, taking payment for caring for these children.

Foster parents represent a unique group. Select individuals become licensed with the intention of becoming adoptive parents, whereas others—at least when they start as foster parents—do not have the intention of building a family through adoption. Others, in the case of kinship parents, which we have discussed, become licensed foster parents and receive additional benefits through the child welfare system for children under their care. Several of the foster parents that I know personally have birth children in the home and have a desire to help vulnerable children. Some do decide to adopt children under their care, whereas others do not. They are dedicated to supporting children who have a wide range of needs.

Therapeutic or special-needs foster parents receive additional training beyond the required core hours. This type of foster care is designed to place a limited number of children (e.g., no more than two) in a home for children with behavioral and/or emotional needs. These children, in essence, require more intense parenting and care. Case managers will identify the type of child that is the best fit for the home; for example, a parent who works well with children with autistic spectrum disorders, or another who cannot care for children who demonstrate sexually maladaptive behavior due to young children in the home. Because there may be multiple medical appointments, one of the foster parents is often not working outside the home (birth parents are invited to join the appointments). Nurses are frequently providers to children with medical needs. Owing to 12-hour shifts, they are able to schedule appointments on their days off. However, finding childcare providers to special needs children when foster parents are at work can be challenging.

In Chapter 2, I briefly described medically fragile children, those patients with the most significant ongoing medical needs (e.g., organ transplant, feeding tube, tracheostomy). Foster parents to these children need even more specialized training and often will go to the hospital to be educated on how to care for the infant or child. The state's Department of Child Services will contract with licensed child placing agencies (LCPAs) to assist in the placement, care, and adoption of children in the child welfare system. The LCPA often requires additional training for foster parents who care for these fragile children. Health care providers, such as APNs, sign medical forms at each appointment, and copies of these forms are provided at least monthly to licensing and state workers. Foster parents log medications and other treatments when administered; this log is also provided to the case managers and state workers. Many children with medical needs have services such as early intervention programs or, at times, a home-based nurse for additional monitoring and care. The state remains the guardian of many medically fragile children.

The National Foster Parent Association (NFPA; www.nfpaonline. org) represents thousands of foster parents and the "over 400,000 children in out-of-home placement in the U.S." (National Foster Parent Association, 2016). The NFPA website offers links to information about conventions and becoming a foster parent.

ASSESSMENT OF CHILD AND ADOLESCENT NEEDS

Several tools exist to assist child welfare agencies in the assessment of children who are placed in out of home (OOH) care. One tool that is being used in various forms in all 50 states is the Child and

Adolescent Needs and Strengths (CANS) tool. The CANS score assists in case planning, directing services, and ties into payment based on an integration of the child/adolescent strengths and needs. There are two primary versions of CANS: one for children ages 0 to 5 years, and one for older children and adolescents ages 6 to 20 years. A CANS is conducted by a certified worker within a specific time limit when the child/adolescent is placed in care. Levels of care are then determined (i.e., levels 0, 1, 2, or 3). Different domains may be assessed as well. For example, there is a Traumatic/Adverse Event Childhood Experiences Domain, CANS Day Treatment, and the Coordination of Complex Care (CANS-CCC) program, all of which have a scoring key and are used as algorithms in assigning care levels (Lyons, 2009). Children under age 16 can be placed in one of four placement types, in increasing levels of restrictiveness: foster care, specialized foster care, group home, and residential treatment (Chor, McClelland, Weiner, Jordan, & Lyons, 2015). APNs may see patients with certain levels of care that are assigned on the basis of various assessments.

CHILDREN IN FOSTER CARE

As previously discussed in Chapter 2, children who are adopted from the foster care system often present with complex physical, behavioral, and psychological needs. The Fostering Connections to Success and Increasing Adoptions Act of 2008 also stipulates more coordination of health care services for these children, regardless of whether they are adopted or not:

SEC. 205. HEALTH OVERSIGHT AND COORDINATION PLAN.

. . . and in consultation with pediatricians, other experts in health care, and experts in and recipients of child welfare services, a plan for the ongoing oversight and coordination of health care services for any child in a foster care placement, which shall ensure a coordinated strategy to identify and respond to the health care needs of children in foster care placements, including mental health and dental health needs, and shall include an outline of—

(i) a schedule for initial and follow-up health screenings that meet reasonable standards of medical practice; (ii) how health needs identified through screenings will be monitored and treated; (iii) how medical information for children in care will be updated and appropriately shared, which may include the development and implementation of an electronic health record; (iv) steps to ensure continuity of health care services, which may include the establishment of a medical home for every child in care; (v) the oversight of prescription medicines; and (vi) how the State actively consults with and involves physicians or other appropriate medical or non-medical professionals in assessing the health and well-being of children in foster care and in determining appropriate medical treatment for the children. . .

These children often have complex needs and may have experienced complex trauma, maltreatment from those who were supposed to nurture, care for, and provide a safe environment. Overall, adolescents in foster care with a history of sexual abuse, aggression, substance abuse, and suicidality, and those who experienced a death or suicide of a parent reported worse health status rankings as compared with those adolescents with best health status (Kools, Paul, Jones, Monasterio, & Norbeck, 2013). If we truly view individuals as holistic beings, then we acknowledge the link between mental health and medical/health care needs. APNs should be alert for those adolescents with these complex mental health issues as they address their overall health care needs.

Emancipation of Youth in Foster Care

Imagine that you have been raised in foster care and long to be independent. Your life has been largely out of your control, and you may have lived with many different foster families through the years. Thoughts of being adopted were long ago placed aside, and now, you cannot wait to finally be free from the system and in control of your life. But what many youth in this situation cannot fully understand are the supports needed for them to succeed in an adult world. Without those services, they remain extremely vulnerable.

Aging out or emancipation of foster youth refers to the end of the legal relationship between the state and the minor, who is under the guardianship of the state, when the youth is at or near the age of majority, usually between 18 and 21 years of age; however, this varies by state (Evan B. Donaldson Adoption Institute, 2011). In 2010, 11% of foster youth were emancipated from foster care; in 5 years, between 2005 and 2010, 167,000 young people left foster care to live independently. The problem is that many of these already at-risk youth are ill-equipped for life outside the foster care system.

The American Academy of Pediatrics (2014) authored the "Moving to Adulthood: A Handout for Youth Aging Out of Foster Care," which includes helpful information in transitioning out of placement (e.g., identification needed, how to sign up for Medicaid, and other valuable resources). APNs can offer this handout, which is available on the Internet, to adolescents and youth adults. Referrals to social service agencies will also be helpful as these youth try to find their way in society as adults.

UNACCOMPANIED REFUGEE MINORS

Children fleeing countries as refugees, entrants, asylees, and victims of trafficking without the benefit of parents or other caregivers enter new countries around the world seeking safety and care. In the United States, the State Department places eligible children into the Unaccompanied Refugee Minors (URM) program to receive refugee foster care services. Lutheran Immigration Refugee Service and the United States Conference of Catholic Bishops are two major voluntary agencies that assist the Office of Refugee Resettlement with the URM program. Peaking in 1985 with 3,828 children, primarily from Southeast Asia, the estimated number of children in the URM program at present is 700. Children in the program are offered the services available to all foster children in the respective states (Office of Refugee Resettlement, 2012). The Survivors of Torture Program provides services for those who have experienced torture in other countries, not uncommon for those seeking refugee status (Office of Refugee Resettlement, 2016).

Little research has been conducted on the needs of URMs; even less so from a health care perspective. Refugee children have been exposed to multiple traumatic events, and some, to torture. They enter the United States without parents or kin, fleeing war and poverty in their native countries. In a case study, Carlson, Cacciatore, and Klimek (2012) tell the story of a boy from Sudan who is able to overcome his trauma, including the death of his half-brother. They identify risk factors (traumatic loss, and chronic, ongoing loss), and protective influences such as individual factors (religiosity, coping skills, school performance, and easy temperament), family protective factors (early, positive family life and positive foster parent relationships), and community protective factors (mentors from school, church, and community organizations; Carlson et al., 2012). Despite the lack of research in health care needs of these children, APNs should be aware of the vulnerabilities of these children and how to build upon the resiliency many of them demonstrate.

ASSISTED REPRODUCTIVE TECHNOLOGY AND EMBRYO DONATIONS

Technology has been used in various forms to both facilitate and discourage conception. Perhaps one of the most common uses of technology employed when couples are faced with infertility is in vitro fertilization (IVF), a method of conceiving a child by fertilizing an egg with sperm outside of the woman's body. During the course of IVF, there are often more embryos created than are used, which are cryopreserved (frozen in liquid nitrogen and stored). Questions surrounding the remaining frozen embryos then become salient: Are the embryos stored indefinitely (there are annual fees to cover the costs of cryopreservation and storage), abandoned, or donated to couples who wish to adopt the embryos? Today, there are approximately 400,000 to 625,000 embryos in cryopreservation (Hoffman et al., 2003; National Embryo Donation Center, 2016).

Thus, a fairly new type of "adoption," embryo donation, has come into being with frozen embryo transfers (FET) being performed into an "adoptive mother" 9 months before the baby is born. With funding from the U.S. Department of Health and Human Services, the National Embryo Donation Academy Reference Manual was created to assist several disciplines: health care professionals, including nurses, as well as social workers, theologians, and policy makers about embryo adoption (Keenan & Little, 2011). The manual is a series of course topics designed to educate various professionals about embryo adoptions. Certain countries have banned embryo adoptions, including China, Italy, and Germany (Keenan & Little, 2011). This technology enters into realms of religious and ethical beliefs about when life begins, and the rights, if any, offered to preimplantation embryos. The vocabulary used in referencing this information stands out. Indeed, some resist the use of the term "embryo adoption," preferring the term "embryo donation." Those who prefer the latter term insist that adoption is an act of transferring parentage of an existing child (see Table 9.1; Keenan & Little, 2011). The paperwork

TABLE 9.1   *How Does Embryo Donation Differ From Traditional Adoption?*

	Embryo Donation	**Traditional Adoption**
	A child born through embryo donation. . .	A child placed through traditional adoption. . .
Genetics	Forever shares the genetic background of their embryo donors.	Forever shares the genetic background of their birth parents.
Medical history	Will always be directly in need of and may be impacted by the past, current, and the ongoing health history of their donors and their donors extended family members.	Will always be directly in need of and may be impacted by the past, current and ongoing health history of their birth parents' extended family members
Future generations	May later give birth to children of their own. These children (and any future generations to come) will also forever be connected to and/or directly influenced by the medical and genetic histories of their parents' donors and extended family.	May later give birth to children of their own. These children (and any future generations to come) will also forever be connected to and/or directly influenced by the medical and genetic histories of their parents' birth parents and extended family.
Genetic siblings	Will always share a genetic and medical relationship to the children of their donors.	Will always share a genetic and medical relationship to the children of their birth parents.

(continued)

TABLE 9.1   *How Does Embryo Donation Differ From Traditional Adoption?*
(*continued*)

Nature versus nurture	May be significantly influenced or impacted by their genetic makeup as scientific evidence suggests that personality makeup, natural abilities, interests/hobbies, and talents are influenced by a combination of both nature and nurture.	May be significantly influenced or impacted by their genetic makeup as scientific evidence suggests that personality makeup, natural abilities, interests/hobbies, and talents are influenced by a combination of both nature and nurture.
In utero experience	Is typically gestated in the womb of the mother that will raise him or her.	Is typically gestated in the womb of the birth mother.
Birth	Will be placed with their nongenetic family before birth and will be born from the mother that will raise him or her.	Will be born from the birth mother who will adoptively place them with another family following birth.
Postbirth	Will be raised by the parents to whom they were born following embryo donation.	Will be raised by the parents with whom they were placed following adoption.
Parents	Will forever, legally and relationally, be the child of the parents that birthed and raised them. However, medical, genetic, and self-identity questions may lead them to having an interest in communicating or one day meeting their embryo donors, as well as any genetic siblings they may have.	Will forever, legally and relationally, be the child of the parents that raised them. However, medical, genetic, and self-identity questions may lead them to having an interest in communicating with or one day meeting their birth parents, as well as any genetic siblings they may have.

Source: Keenan and Little (2011). Reprinted by permission of the authors.

to process the donation may be handled by either a fertility clinic that stores the embryos or an adoption agency. Although many of the ethical implications to embryo donation are fertile ground for debate, this type of "adoption" is increasing. For example, the "intended mother" who carries the embryo is in control of her body and can, thus control her health.

GLOBAL COMMERCIAL SURROGACY

With the rise in infertility rates, the diminished number of available infants for adoption, and the decrease in intercountry adoptions, global commercial surrogacy (GCS) is increasing (Scherman, Misca, Rotabi, & Selman, 2016). This type of "adoption" is distinct from intercountry adoption and traditional surrogacy, but also shares some common elements. Women from outside the United States, currently primarily from India, are hired to carry a child as a surrogate. Estimates are that in India alone, $400 million has been taken in, with 300 clinics designed for this use (Scherman et al., 2016; World of Surrogacy, 2015). A new vocabulary has also arisen with "intended parents/IPs," "commissioning," or "contracting" parents, indicating those who will be the permanent caregivers to the infant once she or he is born. IPs assert there is no exploitation of the surrogate.

Despite this claim, GCS is illegal in Australia, Canada, France, Italy, New Zealand, the UK, and parts of the United States (Scherman et al., 2016). In contrast to private adoption, where there are allowable expenses offered during pregnancy, in GCS the mother is offered money exceeding her expenses. GCS is also available to sexual minority and older parents, which has created continued demand for this type of parenting—demographics that often deny these individuals the ability to adopt a child from another country. The most common type of surrogacy is when the woman is not genetically related to the baby; however, one or both of the IPs are. An embryo is implanted into the surrogate to carry to gestation. This genetic link is a significant motivator for IPs (Scherman et al., 2016).

The media storm following the "Baby Gammy" in 2014 drew attention to the practice of GCS. In essence, an Australian couple hired a surrogate in Thailand to carry twins through gestation for them. When it was discovered that one twin had Down's syndrome, the couple requested that the fetus be aborted. The surrogate refused, and both infants were born; however, the IPs were accused of abandoning the child with Down's, Baby Gammy, a claim they vehemently deny (The Guardian, 2016). To complicate matters, the IP father was convicted of previous sex offenses and had served time in prison for them. Thus, concerns about the vetting process for GCS-intended parents have arisen. APNs may assess infants brought into the United

States through GCS and need to be aware of the ethical, financial, genetic, and health care aspects of this practice.

HUMAN TRAFFICKING

Just the name "human trafficking" harkens back to images of humans being treated as chattel, considered objects to be abused for monetary gain. Today, images have expanded to sex slaves, and children and adolescents treated in degradation, torture, and enslavement. APNs may interact with individuals who are caught in human trafficking, and vulnerable populations are those youth in foster care, those youth who age out of the foster care system (see previous discussion), and those who run away from foster, kinship, and adoptive homes. There are two major types of abuse: sexual exploitation and forced labor. But other types are emerging: forced combat, begging, and petty crimes (United Nations Office on Drugs and Crime [UNODC], 2014). Human trafficking commonly occurs close to home, and there has been an increase in trafficking, especially among young girls. Women are significantly involved, both as victims and as traffickers. Thirty-three percent of victims are children. Yet few perpetrators are reported and convicted (UNODC, 2014). Risk factors include child maltreatment with child protective service/child welfare system involvement, involvement with the juvenile justice system, multiple sexually transmitted infections, pregnancy, substance abuse, behavioral health problems, learning disabilities, living in high-crime areas, and a history of running away from home (Greenbaum, Crawford-Jakubiak, & Committee on Child Abuse and Neglect, 2015).

A new federal law, Preventing Sex Trafficking and Strengthening Families Act (P.L. 113-183/H.R. 4980), was signed by President Obama on September 29, 2014. The act establishes the National Advisory Committee on the Sex Trafficking of Children and Youth in the United States. In summary:

This new law takes important steps forward in protecting and preventing children and youth in foster care from becoming victims of sex trafficking and makes many important improvements to the child welfare system that will help improve outcomes for children and youth in foster care. (p. 1)

New steps allow foster parents to make reasonable and prudent decisions about the child's health and safety and extracurricular activities; ensure children in foster care who are 14 years and older are allowed to participate in their plans; and that children who are aging out of foster care have identification such as birth certificates, social security cards, health insurance information, and a driver's license or state identification (National Conference of State Legislatures, 2016). The law also strengthens reporting of sex trafficking, including data into the Adoption and Foster Care Analysis and Reporting System (AFCARS), and responding to reports of children who are missing (Children's Defense Fund, 2014).

The APN has multiple occasions to interface with victims of human trafficking, and thus opportunities to intervene. The National Human Trafficking Resource Center (NHTRC, 2016a) is a resource for medical professionals who suspect their patient is a victim of human trafficking; it has a variety of tools, literature, and a hotline to post in hallways for patients to see (see Figure 9.1; National Human Trafficking Resource Center [NHTRC], 2016b).

Green (2016) describes strategies for the nurse to employ when approaching patients who may be victimized. First, never ask whether the individual is a victim of human trafficking. They may not understand the term "trafficking" and their companion/abuser may be nearby. Second, the individual may bristle at being referred to as a "victim." Third, try to separate the victim from the trafficker, using examination privacy as a reason to ask them to leave. Fourth, secure an interpreter if the individual does not speak English and insist, if necessary to ensure privacy, that the interpreter has to be approved by the facility. Fifth, be prepared for resistance to help because the individual's emotions may include fear, shame, and helplessness. Ensure that the victim has a medical person with him or her at all times in case the abuser suspects that trafficking is suspected and wants to flee with the patient (Green, 2016). Physical assessment findings often direct the APN to protecting the patient against further abuse (see Table 9.2; Green, 2016).

SUMMARY

This chapter provides an overview of systems and practices that surround adoption and kinship triads. There may be temporal boundaries between these systems and the triads. For example, foster parents may

NHTRC
1-888-373-7888 | NATIONAL
HUMAN TRAFFICKING
RESOURCE CENTER

Human Trafficking Assessment Tool for Medical Professionals

➕ Patient Accesses Medical Services

**Medical
Services are
Provided**

Consider these Red Flags*:
» Someone else is speaking for the patient
» Patient is not aware of his/her location, the current date, or time
» Patient exhibits fear, anxiety, PTSD, submission, or tension
» Patient shows signs of physical/sexual abuse, medical neglect, or torture
» Patient is reluctant to explain his/her injury

If any of these red flags are present, discuss with the patient:

» Speak with the patient alone
» Bring in a social worker or advocate whenever possible
» Use a professional, neutral interpreter if needed

1. Have you been forced to engage in sexual acts for money or favors?
2. Is someone holding your passport or identification documents?
3. Has anyone threatened to hurt you or your family if you leave?
4. Has anyone physically or sexually abused you?
5. Do you have a debt to someone you cannot pay off?
6. Does anyone take all or part of the money you earn?

**If YES to any of the above questions
or if other indicators of human trafficking are present:**
Call the National Human Trafficking Resource Center (NHTRC)
hotline at **1-888-373-7888**
Ask for assistance with assessment and next steps
(following all HIPAA & mandatory reporting regulations)
*The NHTRC Hotline is a confidential hotline, is operated 24/7,
and has access to 200+ languages*

If No to above questions:
Refer to local social services as appropriate

No perceived danger:
The NHTRC can help determine next steps and referrals.

Assessment of Potential Danger
The NHTRC can assist in assessing the current level of danger. Be attentive to the immediate environment for safety concerns and follow hospital protocols if there are safety threats. Questions to consider:
» Is the trafficker present?
» What does the patient believe will happen if they do not return?
» Does the patient believe anyone else (including family) is in danger?
» Is the patient a minor?

Local Resources:
Refer to existing community resources included in a response protocol as needed, as the NHTRC may not have all local referrals in their database. If there is no current response protocol in place, consider establishing one.

If there is perceived danger and the patient wants help:
Discuss with the Hotline next steps. You may need to involve law enforcement for victim safety. The NHTRC can assist in determining sensitive law enforcement contacts.

*For more red flags and indicators see the NHTRC's Comprehensive Assessment Tool and Identifying Victims of Human Trafficking document for healthcare providers.

Report Online or Access Resources & Referrals: www.traffickingresourcecenter.org
Call: 1-888-373-7888 (24/7)   **Email:** nhtrc@polarisproject.org

This publication was made possible in part through Grant Number 90ZV0102 from the Anti-Trafficking in Persons Division, Office of Refugee Resettlement, U.S. Department of Health and Human Services (HHS). Its contents are solely the responsibility of the authors and do not necessarily represent the official views of the Anti-Trafficking in Persons Division, Office of Refugee Resettlement, or HHS.

FIGURE 9.1   *Human trafficking assessment tool for medical professionals.*

TABLE 9.2 *Common Assessment Findings Associated With Human Trafficking*

Suspect your patient may be a trafficking victim if your assessment reveals the findings listed below. Also, laboratory tests may indicate sexually transmitted infections, dehydration, untreated diabetes, and positive drug screens.

Body System	Findings
Skin	☐ Signs of trauma ☐ Brands or tattoos ☐ Bruising ☐ Scars ☐ Lacerations ☐ Infestations (Note: Signs of abuse that leave a mark typically are in low-visibility areas, such as the lower back.)
Reproductive tract	☐ Genital mutilation or scarring ☐ Fistulas ☐ Signs of multiple terminated pregnancies ☐ Vaginal or anal trauma ☐ Pelvic inflammatory disease
Musculoskeletal system	☐ Poorly healed fractures ☐ Signs of repeated strains ☐ Abnormal gait in a younger person
Respiratory system	☐ Tuberculosis infection ☐ Untreated asthma or bronchitis
Psychosocial status	☐ Exaggerated startle response ☐ Panic or anxiety ☐ Flat affect ☐ Withdrawal or refusal to engage ☐ Signs of drug or alcohol abuse or withdrawal

Source: Green (2016). Reprinted by permission.

transition into adoptive parents as they decide to provide permanent homes for children under their care. Other emerging practices such as embryo donations, emerging special groups such as URM, and surrogates from developing nations, provide glimpses into the influences of technology, money, and war, and how complex our world is becoming. Last, human trafficking and the victimization of children and adolescents provide scenarios where the legal system and health care meet. In each situation, opportunities are presented for APNs to deliver humane, patient-centered, informed care.

CHAPTER HIGHLIGHTS

☐ Foster care parents and children are unique groups that create families, on both short- and long-term bases. Many foster care parents will care for children for varying lengths of time, sometimes many years without legally adopting them. Federal legislation has mandated that children who are aging out now have a coordinated service plan in place.

☐ A small but significant number of children immigrate to the United States, fleeing war and poverty in their home countries. These children are in special foster care called the Unaccompanied Refugee Minors program.

☐ Assisted embryo donations are increasing in number as a viable form of parenting. However, there are important differences between embryo donation and traditional adoption.

☐ Commercial surrogacy is emerging as a new practice because of globalization, the demand for infants, the increase in infertility rates, and the decrease in intercountry adoption.

☐ Children and adolescents in nontraditional families, including the foster care system, and kinship and adoptive families, are vulnerable to human trafficking. This heinous victimization calls for APNs in urgent, acute, and primary care settings to be vigilant in identifying common signs and symptoms of individuals who are victims of human trafficking.

Questions for Reflection

Following are a few questions to reflect upon. You can use these to start a journal for yourself or in a classroom discussion with peers and the instructor.

1. When you hear the words "foster child," what are your immediate thoughts, emotions, overall reactions? Are these based on

personal or professional experiences, or, in general, on how our society views children in the public welfare system?

2. In what ways are embryo donation truly adoption? In what ways does it differ? Are the individuals that donate embryos similar to birth parents? How does this technology make us question certain assumptions we hold about when human life begins?

3. If you have ever cared for a person who was involved in human trafficking, reflect upon the care you rendered. Did it involve a person who is responsible for the suffering of others? What were the circumstances? Were you satisfied with your actions as an APN? What would you have done differently, if anything? How did you process this experience?

References

American Academy of Pediatrics. (2014). Moving to adulthood: A handout for youth aging out of foster care. Retrieved from www.aap.org/en-us/advocacy-and-policy/aap-health-initiatives/healthy-foster-care-america/Documents/AgingOut%20FINAL.pdf

Carlson, B. E., Cacciatore, J., & Klimek, B. (2012). A risk and resilience perspective on unaccompanied refugee minors. *Social Work, 57*(3), 259–269. doi:10.1093/sw/sws003

Children's Defense Fund. (2014). *Preventing Sex Trafficking and Strengthening Families Act (H.R. 4980).* Washington, DC: Author. Retrieved from www.childrensdefense.org/library/data/fact-sheet-on-hr-4980.pdf

Chor, K. H., McClelland, G. M., Weiner, D. A., Jordan, N., & Lyons, J. S. (2015). Out-of-home placement decision-making and outcomes in child welfare: A longitudinal study. *Administration and Policy in Mental Health and Mental Health Services Research, 42*(10), 70–86. doi:10.1007/s10488-014-0545-5

Evan B. Donaldson Adoption Institute. (2011). *Never too old: Achieving permanency and sustaining connections for older youth in foster care.* New York, NY: Author.

Green, C. (2016). Human trafficking: Preparing for a unique patient population. *American Nurse Today, 11*(1), 9–12.

Greenbaum, J., Crawford-Jakubiak, J. E., & Committee on Child Abuse and Neglect. (2015). Child sex trafficking and commercial sexual exploitation: Health care needs of victims. *Pediatrics, 135*(3), 566–574. doi:10.1542/peds.2014-4138

The Guardian. (2016, April 14). *Baby Gammy's twin can stay with Australian couple despite father's child sex offenses.* Retrieved from www.theguardian .com/lifeandstyle/2016/apr/14/baby-gammys-twin-sister-stays-with -western-australian-couple-court-orders

Hoffman, D. I., Zellman, G. L., Fair, C. C., Mayer, J. F., Zeitz, J. G., Gibbons, W. E., & Turner, T. G. in association with The Society for Assisted Reproductive Technology & RAND. (2003). Cryopreserved embryos in the United States and their availability for research. *Fertility and Sterility, 79*(5), 1063–1069. doi:10.1016/S0015-0282(03)00172-9

Keenan, J., & Little, K. (2011). *The National Embryo Donation Academy reference manual.* Knoxville, TN: National Embryo Donation Academy. Retrieved from www.embryodonation.org/wp-content/uploads/2015/01/ webManual.pdf

Kools, S., Paul, S. M., Jones, R., Monasterio, E., & Norbeck, J. (2013). Health profiles of adolescents in foster care. *Journal of Pediatric Nursing, 28*, 213–222. doi:10.1016/j.pedn.2012.08.010

Lyons, J. S. (2009). *Communimetrics: A communication theory of measurement in human service settings.* New York, NY: Springer Publishing.

National Conference of State Legislatures. (2016). *Preventing Sex Trafficking and Strengthening Families Act of 2014.* Retrieved from www.ncsl .org/research/human-services/preventing-sex-trafficking-and -strengthening-families-act-of-2014.aspx

National Embryo Donation Center. (2016). About us. Retrieved from www .embryodonation.org

National Foster Parent Association. (2016). The national voice of foster parents. Retrieved from nfpaonline.org/

National Human Trafficking Resource Center. (2016a). What is human trafficking? Retrieved from traffickingresourcecenter.org/

National Human Trafficking Resource Center. (2016b). Human trafficking assessment for medical personnel. Retrieved from trafficking resourcecenter.org/resources/human-trafficking-assessment-medical -professionals

Office of Refugee Resettlement. (2012). Unaccompanied refugee minors. Retrieved from www.acf.hhs.gov/programs/orr/resource/unaccompanied -refugee-minors

Office of Refugee Resettlement. (2016). Survivors of torture program. Retrieved from www.acf.hhs.gov/programs/orr/programs/survivors-of-torture

Scherman, R., Misca, G., Rotabi, K., & Selman, P. (2016). Global commercial surrogacy and international adoption: Parallels and differences. *Adoption & Fostering, 40*(1), 20–35. doi:10.1177/0308575915626376

United Nations Office on Drugs and Crime. (2014). *Global report on trafficking in persons* (United Nations Publication, Sales No. E.14.V.10). New York, NY: United Nations Publication.

World of Surrogacy. (2015). Five things you should know about surrogacy. Retrieved from www.worldofsurrogacy.com/surrogacy/

III

Position Statement Regarding Adoption and Kinship Nursing

10

Conclusions and Future Directions

□ □ □ □

PURPOSE OF THIS CHAPTER

The purpose of this final chapter is to provide a synthesis of information built on the previous chapters, as well as to offer a potential map for our future endeavors as a nursing profession. As I mentioned in the beginning of this book, nurses are important caregivers to adoptive and kinship triads, yet as a profession, we lack standards of care for these patients. I propose a subspecialty designation through the American Nurses Association (ANA), with scope and standards of practice for Adoption and Kinship Nursing. These standards of practice will guide nurses at the baccalaureate and advanced practice levels to provide patient-centered, quality care to members of these triads. Such standards will recognize the unique body of knowledge that exists in providing care to children and all of their parents (birth, adoptive, and kinship).

Learning Objectives

At the completion of the chapter, the reader will be able to:

1. Summarize the multifaceted roles advanced practice nurses (APNs) have in caring for members of the adoptive and kinship triads
2. Analyze the nursing profession's interface with medical organizations, such as the American Academy of Pediatrics (AAP) and the American College of Obstetrics and Gynecologists (ACOG), in providing care

3. Understand the need for the formation of scope and standards of practice for adoption and kinship nursing
4. Synthesize the ANA (2015) *Code of Ethics* with the provision of APN care to adoptive and kinship families

THE POWERFUL INFLUENCE OF NURSING CARE

This clinical guide has forwarded the principle that advanced practice nurses (APNs) and other nurses are located in key positions to support adoptive and kinship triads. Now, we understand more clearly what to assess for and the best practices on intervening. In summary,

> One primary responsibility of the nurse is to be knowledgeable about sound child placement practices, legal controls governing relinquishment and adoption, and community resources which provide services for those who plan to adopt a child or to place a child for adoption. . . . A second primary responsibility of the nurse is to refer those needing help to that community resource which can provide the direct service needed. (p. 14)

This quote was taken from the Maternal-Child-Health Inter Divisional Council of Colorado League for Nursing (1961); the report was generated in response to data collected from 49 nurses and the care based on various situations surrounding relinquishment. The report describes how "2/3 either did not handle the problem, or handled it in such a way which, if viewed from the parent's standpoint could only be considered vague, misleading or confusing" (p. 2). My sincere hope is that after reading this guide, this statement does not apply to you and that together we can correct the vague, misleading, and confusing messages that may have been conveyed to adoptive- and kinship-related families.

The adoption community and our society have traveled far from the austere orphan houses of the early 1900s (see Exhibit 10.1). I believe with informed nursing care, we can travel even greater distances to provide quality, patient-centered care to members of the adoptive and kinship triads.

EXHIBIT 10.1
ORPHAN HOME, ADDISON, ILLINOIS, 1903

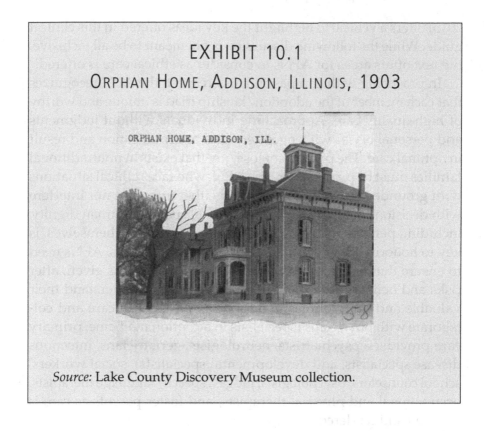

ORPHAN HOME, ADDISON, ILL.

Source: Lake County Discovery Museum collection.

NEXT STEPS FOR THE NURSING PROFESSION: SCOPE AND STANDARDS OF PRACTICE

The Graduate Level Quality and Safety Education for Nurses (QSEN; American Association of Colleges of Nursing [AACN], 2012) guidance provided a framework in this clinical guide. Each of the six areas was discussed (quality improvement, safety, teamwork and collaboration, patient-centered care, evidence-based practice, and informatics) as it applied to nursing care of the adoptive and kinship triads. In addition to these areas, a discussion of the ANA's scope and standards of practice and the *Code of Ethics for Nurses with Interpretive Statements* (*Code of Ethics*; ANA, 2015) will be the springboards and anchors to working groups devoted to generating, refining, and ultimately disseminating these standards of practice. The *Code of Ethics* (ANA,

2015) offers a vehicle to highlight the key ideas offered in this clinical guide. While the following discussion is not meant to be all inclusive, the text offers areas for APNs to consider as ethical care is offered.

In practicing with compassion and respect, the APN recognizes that each member of the adoption/kinship triad is unique and worthy of high-quality care. Approaching individuals without judgments and personal biases will engender open communication and result in optimal care. The paradox of loss/joy that exists in nontraditional families must be processed by the APN, who faces ethical situations with grounded personal values that neither influence nor interfere with decisions made by triad members. Respecting human dignity, including persons who may not be able to speak for themselves, is key to honoring triad and nontraditional relationships. APNs need to ensure that informed consent, free from coercion, is given, after risks and benefits are presented. Nurses need to understand their valuable and unique roles in adoption and kinship care and collaborate with physicians (specialists in adoption medicine, primary care providers, psychiatrists, neurologists, geriatricians, infectious disease specialists, and developmental specialists), social workers, school counselors, psychologists, judges, speech/language therapists, occupational and physical therapists, and foster parents as care is planned and rendered.

The APN's commitment to the patient may take many forms, and as time progresses, the "patient" may change. The triad itself, or the family unit including nuclear and extended families, or generations of a family may be seen as the patient. APNs will need to balance different patient interests, using ethical principles as guides (e.g., fidelity, justice, informed consent, beneficence). Depending on the clinical setting, APNs will need to identify whether any conflict of interest or professional boundaries skew care offered to triad members. Nurses are often members of these triads, and personal experiences must be tempered given the unique presentations of patients.

As we have discussed, confidentiality in adoption is significantly affected by state laws related to sealing of adoption records, which may include health and medical histories. Relinquishment of the child also requires nurses to adhere to the Health Insurance Portability and Accountability Act of 1996 (HIPAA). There's more than health information at stake; there's a life-altering decision that has been made by birth parents to implement an adoption plan. Respecting that plan requires discretion and following the law. The stigma attached to kinship parenting also requires APNs' discretion and adherence to HIPAA. APNs must be willing to act on instances when unethical, illegal, or immoral acts are committed. Advocacy for patients in vulnerable, powerless positions must prevent or address victimization by others in their environments. Nurses must also prevent intended or unintended harm by those in the adoption community whose self-interests threaten to supersede the interests of the patient. Nurses who offer care to the adoptive and kinship triads need to be prepared to offer such health management. Delineation of scope of practice and standards of care are needed to design curricula and continuing education to increase nurses' competence in adoption and kinship care.

APNs can no longer see themselves as supplements to the social worker in caring for adoption and kinship families, but as much-needed providers with the authority, accountability, and responsibility to render such care. Being adoption informed and applying adoption- and kinship-specific knowledge to patients across the life span require an acceptance of such authority. The assessment, diagnoses, goals, interventions, and evaluation of nursing care and nursing orders specific to these groups of patients require that APNs evaluate their own competence to deliver safe, high-quality, patient-centered care.

Nurses may strongly identify with members of the adoption and kinship triads and often are members themselves. Their sense of wholeness may be enhanced or challenged when faced with birth parents' decisions to make an adoption plan, when an adoptive or kinship parent assumes the caregiver role to a child, and when a child/adolescent/adult struggles to process his or her relinquishment. Recognizing emotional, spiritual, psychological, and social triggers that may be created through caring for these families is important as APNs promote their own sense of well-being.

Unlike many clinical areas that physically lend themselves to being confined to specific environments—for example, cardiovascular nursing—individuals who are members of adoption and kinship families exist across many clinical settings. The macro environment that influences adoption and kinship is federal legislation, then state statues, followed by specific organizations that form networks comprising health care and adoption/kinship workers. However, the environment as it pertains to adoption and kinship care is fluid and as we have seen throughout this guide, these groups of individuals exist in multiple health care settings and present across the life span with multifaceted health care needs.

Genetics/genomics nursing is similar to adoption/kinship families in that patients present in myriad settings and require vastly different counseling and care. Thus, what we do as APNs and in our practice becomes an environment in itself, and our virtues and obligations become the operating principles and nonphysical boundaries of the environment. For example, how a school nurse assists a pregnant teenager, how an A-GNP assesses an older kinship parent for mal-nutrition in a primary care setting, and how a PNP orders laboratory work to assess for iron levels in a newly adopted child from Ethiopia are all instances wherein APNs' moral virtues and obligations create the foundation of an ethical environment.

Nurse scholars have made significant contributions to the science of adoption and kinship care (see the work of Fontenot, Kelley, Musil, McGuinness, Narad-Mason, and Sandelowski). Many additional "grey" literature pieces exist in the archives as theses and dissertations conducted by graduate nursing students. Yet, we have not professionally integrated this specialized care as an object of study and nursing education, often handing it off instead to social workers and psychologists. I am part of a working group of a national adoption organization that strives to disseminate best practices uncovered in research. In one conversation, we discussed several articles that had recently been published, and the group was trying to decide which ones we thought should be included in an abbreviated summary in a national newsletter published by a large adoption organization. I voted for the health-related studies, but the others pointed out that they were not especially helpful to the audience, who were primarily social workers, adoption staff members, and psychologists. And they were exactly right—the audience was not health care professionals. This experience solidified my goal of creating a specialized area of nursing, adoption and kinship nursing, so that scholarly information can be generated, shared, and become evidence-based practices in health care settings.

We are also striving to be partners in research teams that examine variables in adoption and kinship families. My goal is for research teams to understand that nurses, and the insights and expertise we bring, are invaluable collaborators. Policy is another area we can bring forward to help ensure that each member of the triad's rights are protected and the best interest of the child is reflected in the actions of the professionals around him or her.

Vulnerable families such as those that are created as a result of adoption and kinship placement have special, yet universal, health needs. APNs are well placed to meet these needs because we view the client/person/patient in a whole way. We do not merely diagnose, treat, and manage; we place health and well-being in an informed context, including developmental (pediatric, adult, and older adult) and environmental (health disparities and issues of parity). We understand the global implications of intercountry adoptions and the politics of gender both domestically and across the globe. Children who have experienced maltreatment and trauma are some of the most vulnerable clients that APNs will ever encounter. By understanding trauma, health disparities, human trafficking, and the prevalence of food insecurity, APNs will be able to suspend judgments on diagnoses when symptoms overlap, thereby avoiding premature and erroneous conclusions, and instead, forwarding a treatment plan that is effective and safe.

Having received my first nursing license at the age of 19, I was not—could not—appreciate the beauty of nursing and what it contributes to health care and the well-being of people. Through diverse professional positions, I have worked alongside many teams, and even taught business communication in a Top Ten business school. What I encountered was a stark contrast between the motivations of the business and nursing students. Nursing students study in order to prepare themselves to help people. What they may not understand is that helping people is being part of a collective body that represents the values of the profession. Nursing is viewed as trustworthy and ethical. Although the media juxtaposes nurses as sexual beings or addicts, it also portrays us in a heroic fashion (Hurricane Katrina and other natural disasters). Trust, heroism, advocacy, and risk taking are intrinsic to taking care of individuals whose lives are touched by adoption or kinship. APNs' ability to affect the social justice surrounding adoption and kinship families has been present for many years, although in silos of practice, education, and research. The American Academy of Pediatrics (AAP) and the

American College of Obstetrics and Gynecologists (ACOG) help us to see what collective thought and action brings to professions and society as a whole. Nurses must articulate their contributions to caring for these unique populations and fill the gaps that other health care professions leave—a gap that, in my opinion, can only be filled by nurses. My hope is that with this clinical guide, we can open formal conversations to endorse this specialty area of nursing and advanced practice.

CONCLUDING THOUGHTS

This clinical guide began with a personal narrative about a young student nurse and the impression that a foster family made on her. I would like to conclude with a more recent narrative that I think symbolizes the essence of many nontraditional families. At a kinship parenting class that I was co-facilitating, one parent spoke up and described extremely challenging behaviors she was trying to understand from her 5-year-old grandson. She became tearful as she described what he had experienced and witnessed, and the maltreatment that had created behaviors she could not cope with. While the class for the parents was in session, the children had been working on a craft, supervised by student nurses. Then they rejoined their kinship parents during the break. The little boy, skinny with close cropped hair and tired eyes, walked up to his grandmother and handed her a thin, white, paper crown that had been carefully taped together. The crown was fragile and yet strong because of how he had strategically taped the pieces together. She looked at it for a second, not knowing what it was, then smiled and placed it on her head. She wore it for the rest of the class and each time I looked at her, my eyes went upward and saw that white crown and knew that to this boy, despite what he had endured and because of what she was trying to give him, she was very special. She was his queen.

CHAPTER HIGHLIGHTS

☐ Nursing has historically been involved with caring for adoption and kinship families; nonetheless, we have yet to articulate this care through systematic efforts in education, practice, and research.

☐ Scope and standards of practice for adoption and kinship nursing should be developed in order to formally articulate the care we render to these populations.

Questions for Reflection

Following are a few questions to reflect upon. You can use these to start a journal for yourself or in a classroom discussion with peers and the instructor.

1. What unique body of knowledge does the profession of nursing possess to support a subspecialty area of adoption and kinship nursing?
2. What would you include in scope and standards of practice for nurses interested in working with adoption and kinship triads?
3. How should the profession forward policies that support adoption and kinship families?

References

American Association of Colleges of Nursing. (2012). *Graduate-level QSEN competencies: Knowledge, skills, and attitudes.* Washington, DC: Author. Retrieved from www.aacn.nche.edu/faculty/qsen/competencies.pdf

American Nurses Association (2015). *Code of ethics for nursing with interpretive statements.* Silver Spring, MD: Author.

Maternal-Child-Health Inter Divisional Council of Colorado League for Nursing. (1961). *The role of the nurse in relinquishments and adoptions in Colorado: 1961.* Wheat Ridge, CO: Colorado League for Nursing.

Glossary

□ □ □ □

Acute trauma: Usually considered a one-time traumatic eEvent that is experienced or witnessed. Examples include physical or sexual assault or witnessing violence.

Adopters: A term for adoptive parents; considered by some to have a negative connotation.

Adoption: A legal process whereby a nonbiological parent assumes the care for a child and confers all the rights on that child, including heritable rights as any other child would receive. Birth parents must have parental rights terminated in order for adoption to occur.

Adoption agency: A nonprofit or for-profit business, licensed by the state(s) in which it operates, and arranges placement of children with adoptive parents.

Adoption disclosures: The release of information to an adopted person. Official disclosures may be in the form of previously state-sealed documents; informal disclosures may be in the form of conversations between adoptive parents and their children related to the adoption.

Adoption/kinship-competent or adoption/kinship-informed provider: Health care providers and other professionals who interact with adoption and kinship triads and understand the unique dynamics and needs of these groups.

Adoption facilitator: Is a third party that acts as a middleman in arranging an independent adoption, usually for a fee. Adoption attorneys and psychotherapists may act as facilitators when working with prospective adoptive parents and birth parents.

Adoption attorney: A lawyer who assists in the adoption of a child. This individual may take various roles in the adoption process, from facilitator to an individual who assists in the finalization of the adoption.

Adoptive parent: An individual who becomes the legal parent of a child who is not genetically linked to them. Parentage to adopted children is identical to that of biological children.

Adoption plan: A plan put in place by one or both birth parents with the intention of placing the child with adoptive parents. Such plans may specify whether the adoption will be open, semiopen, or closed.

Adoption subsidy/assistance: Financial assistance given to parents who adopt children with special needs. The assistance will help to cover expenses related to medical services, therapy, and other maintenance costs.

Adoption triad or triangle: The parties involved in an adoptive family, which include the child, the birth parent, and the adoptive parent.

Aging out or emancipation: Within the context of foster care, aging out, or emancipation, refers to the end of the legal relationship between the state and the minor who is under the guardianship of the state when the youth is at or near the age of majority, usually between 18 and 21 years of age. However, this age varies by state.

Birth/biological parent: An individual who gave birth to or helped conceive a child and is, therefore, genetically linked to the child. A birth parent may be unable to or unwilling to care for a child and releases the child into the care of adoptive, kinship, or foster parents.

Chronic trauma: Ongoing, long-standing, or multiple traumatic experiences and/or events such as neglect or physical and sexual abuse.

Closed/confidential/traditional adoption: Adoptions in which the biological parent(s)' identity is sealed at the time of relinquishment; no contact is planned between the birth parent, the child, and the adoptive parents.

Complex trauma: Multiple, severe, profound traumatic experiences and events that may be pervasive and involve family members.

Court-appointed special advocate (CASA) volunteer: An individual appointed by the judge in cases of child abuse and neglect; this volunteer will advocate for the interests of the child and work to ensure that the child does not get lost in the legal and social service systems.

Crisis pregnancy: A pregnancy that is unplanned and creates a crisis for the woman and her partner.

Displacement: Refers to situations when adopted children are placed in foster care or in other living situations, such as group homes.

Disrupted adoption: Occurs when the child, who has been placed in the adoptive home but before the adoption has been legally finalized, is removed from the home. The child is placed either into foster care or with new adoptive parents.

Dissolution of adoption: An adoption that legally ends after finalization. The child is placed either into foster care or with new adoptive parents.

Failed adoption: An adoption plan that is not completed. This may be for a number of reasons, including birth parents altering the plan, the death of the child, or other circumstances that prevent the infant/child from being received by adoptive parents. Disrupted and dissolved adoptions are also considered failed adoptions.

Fictive kin: Individuals involved in raising children who are related neither by blood nor by marriage to the child. Usually they are close family friends.

First/birth parent: Another term for birth parent; the term is used to indicate that this parent was the first parent to the infant/child.

Foster care: Care of a child, usually arranged through government or con-tracted social service agencies, including foster family homes, relative foster care, and group home care. The United States and some countries that send children for intercountry adoption use the foster care system to provide a family living situation for children whose parents are unable to do so.

Gestational surrogate versus traditional surrogate: In both types of sur-rogacy, a woman carries a child through gestation; however, in gestational surrogacy, the surrogate is not genetically linked to the infant. In contrast, the woman in traditional surrogacy has a genetic tie to the offspring through donating her egg to the embryo.

Grandfamilies: Kinship families who are headed by grandparents or other close family members and friends.

Hague Convention: Hague Convention on the Protection of Children and Co-operation in Respect of Intercountry Adoption (Hague Convention) is an international treaty with the purpose of protecting child rights, decreas-ing human trafficking, and ensuring there is no conflict of interest in those who are arranging adoptions.

Independent adoptions: Adoptions that occur without the services of an adoption agency; these are arranged between the birth and the adoptive parents. Adoption attorneys may also be involved.

Kinship caregivers/parents: Raising of the child by grandparents and other close family members and friends. These families have a variety of typolo-gies and connections with the child welfare system.

Kinship triad or triangle: The parties involved in a kinship family, which include: the child, the birth parent, and the kinship parent, usually a grandparent.

Medical home: Also known as a patient-centered medical home, it is headed by a health care provider with the intention of delivering continuous, comprehensive, and coordinated medical care.

Open adoption: An arrangement that includes contact between the birth and the adoptive parents. Open adoption may include varying levels of contact, from letters to face-to-face visits, and may be accomplished with the help of a third party.

Patient-centered care: Care that is individualized to the patient, taking into consideration their preferences, wants, and needs. It is a philosophy that is reflected in partnership between the provider, and the patient and family, and is guided by the patient values (whenever this is appropriate).

Postadoption contact agreement/cooperative adoption agreement: An arrangement agreed upon by the birth and adoptive parents, which can range from an informal agreement to a legal contract. This agreement outlines future contact with birth families and others who have an established relationship with the child so that expectations can be defined.

Putative father: A man who claims to be or who is alleged to be the father of a child with a woman whom he is not married to at the time of the infant's birth.

Receiving country: A country that receives children from other countries with the goal of placing them in adoptive homes.

Relative placement: Placement of a child in the care of a relative through the foster care system. Relatives may include grandparents, aunts, uncles, adult siblings, and cousins. Some states also consider tribal members as relatives.

Sending country: Designation for countries that send children to receiving nations, such as the United States. Reputable adoption agencies will strive to place orphans within their country of origin rather than sending them abroad to be adopted.

Therapeutic foster care: Placement of children with specific needs (physical, behavioral, and medical) in foster homes with specially trained foster parents. These children usually require more intensive care than children in typical foster placements.

Unnecessary adoptions: Adoptions that occur as a result of financial or resource-related issues in a birth parent's life. Situations in which, if proper resources were allocated, the need to adopt would no longer exist.

Recommended Reading

□ □ □ □

Brodzinsky, D. M., & Palacios, J. (Eds.). (2005). *Psychological issues in adoption: Research and practice.* Westport, CT: Praeger Publishers.

Conn, P. (2013). *Adoption: A brief social and cultural history.* New York, NY: Palgrave Macmillan.

Eldridge, S. (1999). *Twenty things adopted kids wish their adoptive parents knew.* New York, NY: Dell Publishing.

Foli, K. J., & Thompson, J. R. (2004). *The post-adoption blues: Overcoming the unforeseen challenges of adoption.* Emmaus, PA: Rodale.

Keck, G., & Kupecky, R. (2009a). *Adopting the hurt child: Hope for families with special-needs kids: A guide for parents and professionals.* Colorado Springs, CO: NavPress.

Keck, G., & Kupecky, R. (2009b). *Parenting the hurt child: Helping adoptive families heal and grow.* Colorado Springs, CO: NavPress.

Mason, P. W., Johnson, D. E., & Prock, L. A. (Eds.). (2014). *Adoption medicine.* Elk Grove Village, IL: American Academy of Pediatrics.

Melosh, B. (2002). *Strangers and kin: The American way of adoption.* Cambridge, MA: Harvard University Press.

Phagan-Hansel, K. (Ed.). (2012). *The foster parenting toolbox: A practical, hands-on approach to parenting children in foster care.* Warren, NJ: EMK Press.

Phagan-Hansel, K. (Ed.). (2015). *The kinship parenting toolbox: A unique guide for the kinship care parenting journey.* Warren, NJ: EMK Press.

Purvis, K. B., Cross, D. R., & Lyons Sunshine, W. (2007). *The connected child: Bring hope and healing to your adoptive family.* New York, NY: McGraw-Hill.

Roorda, R. (2000). *In their own voices: Transracial adoptees tell their stories.* New York, NY: Columbia University Press.

Roorda, R. (2015). *In their voices: Black Americans on transracial adoption.* New York, NY: Columbia University Press.

Index

□ □ □ □

Printed in the United States
By Bookmasters